Instructor's Manual with Test Bank for

NURSING IN
TODAY'S WORLD

Challenges, Issues, and Trends

Fifth Edition

Janice Rider Ellis, PhD, RN
Professor and Director of Nursing Education
Shoreline Community College
Seattle, Washington

Celia Love Hartley, MN, RN
Professor and Chairperson, Allied Health
Director, Nursing Programs
College of the Desert
Palm Desert, California

Instructor's Manual with Test Bank for

NURSING IN TODAY'S WORLD

Challenges, Issues, and Trends

Fifth Edition

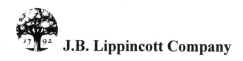

J.B. Lippincott Company

Acquisitions Editor: Margaret Belcher, RN, BSN
Coordinating Editorial Assistant: Emily A. Cotlier
Ancillary Coordinator: Doris S. Wray
Keyboarder/Typist: Rose M. Jones
Copy editing: Joy R. Perry
Compositor: Richard G. Hartley
Printer/Binder: R.R. Donnelly, Crawfordsville

Fifth Edition

6 5 4 3 2 1

0-397-55181-9

Any procedure or practice described in this book should be applied by the health-care practitioner under appropriate supervision in accordance with professional standards of care used with regard to the unique circumstances that apply in each practice situation. Care has been taken to confirm the accuracy of information presented and to describe generally accepted practices. However, the authors, editors, and publisher cannot accept any responsibility for errors or omissions or for any consequences from application of information in this book and make no warranty express or implied, with respect to the contents of this book.

Every effort has been made to ensure drug selections and dosages are in accordance with current recommendations and practice. Because of ongoing research, changes in government regulations and the constant flow of information on drug therapy, reactions and interactions, the reader is cautioned to check the package insert for each drug for indications, dosages, warnings, and precautions, particularly if the drug is new or infrequently used.

Preface

Any program of learning pursued by today's nursing students would be incomplete without the inclusion of information about the profession itself. It is critical that nurses have an understanding of the circumstances and events that have shaped the profession of nursing as we know it. We also recognize that nursing curricula must place strong emphasis on critical decision making in a clinically oriented setting while concomitantly focusing on the skillful performance of numerous nursing procedures. Because of the time that must be devoted to clinically oriented courses, it is our concern that the "issues" related to nursing may take a back seat in curriculum development and emphasis. Our goal in developing this instructor's manual is to facilitate the instruction and evaluation of the content related to the profession itself, to be used in conjunction with the textbook *Nursing in Today's World: Challenges, Issues and Trends.*

Each chapter in this manual corresponds with a chapter in the textbook. A statement of purpose provides a discussion of the major content covered in the chapter. The objectives repeat those included at the beginning of each textbook chapter and are intended to provide ready reference for the instructor. The significant terminology section identifies words or phrases that the student should understand after studying the chapter content. In some instances this is a very short list, in other cases rather long, depending on the material discussed. For example, one would naturally expect a longer terminology list for chapters related to legal implications or collective bargaining in nursing.

A variety of test situations appear next in each chapter. They are developed in several different formats so that the instructor may select those that best meet the needs of a particular program. In some instances there are more of one type of question than another; however, there are a number of test questions provided for each chapter.

With this edition we have added a section of questions devoted to critical thinking activities. Critical thinking, as we use it here, is the process by which an individual analyzes and synthesizes material from multiple sources from an evaluative viewpoint. Logically completed it results in a clearer, more precise, more significant and depthful answer that has looked analytically at all possibilities before selecting the best. We see this process as tantamount to good nursing practice today; thus, we provide situations that will give students the opportunity to practice the skill.

The discussion/essay questions can be used in a number of ways. First, they can be used to direct the discussion that would occur in a seminar-format class. In this sense, they can also be used as preparation for a "credit-by-examination" test if an instructor deems it appropriate to make that option available to students. Questions selected from this section might also be used appropriately for take-home finals or as regular midterm or end-of-the-term examinations. You will notice that each question is keyed to a particular objective of the chapter. This is intended to facilitate "teaching by objectives" and "testing by objectives." It is also intended to assist those who teach in programs where the content is integrated. Thus, objectives related to specific topics can be selected and corresponding test questions readily identified.

The matching questions are offered as yet another form of evaluating learning. They might be used by the students as a study guide or incorporated into the general testing or content.

Multiple-choice and true-false questions can be used similarly. You will note that there are often several questions that address a particular objective or, more specifically, a particular concept. This is intended to allow the instructor to select a wording that best matches his or her class emphasis. It also allows for the development of different, yet equivalent, examinations if the course is taught each term. Some of the questions are very basic and therefore can be used as a pretest at the beginning of each class if desired. This form of questioning can be readily adapted to grading machines. The possible choices can also be altered to reflect the emphasis developed in a particular course.

We hope this manual will assist and facilitate your instruction. As with the major textbook, we welcome your suggestions for change or improvement.

Janice Rider Ellis, RN, PhD
Celia Love Hartley, RN, MN

Table of Contents

1 | Nursing as a Developing Profession

Purpose

Chapter 1 reviews the development of nursing as a profession and distinguishes it from medicine. It outlines the characteristics of a profession and discusses the challenges offered to nursing with regard to these characteristics. The chapter reviews the practice of medicine and the practice of nursing, to the extent that it existed, in the major early cultures. The historical image of nursing is reviewed and present-day aspects of nursing's image are scrutinized. The life of Florence Nightingale is briefly discussed, with emphasis on the ways in which she influenced the development of nursing as a profession. The chapter concludes with a discussion of the major studies conducted about nurses and nursing and outlines why they were undertaken; further, it discusses the major recommendations of each study.

Objectives

1. *Discuss the reasons the profession has had difficulty defining nursing.*

2. *Give a definition of nursing and identify a theorist who defines nursing similarly.*

3. *Using the formal characteristics provided, determine whether you believe nursing is a profession.*

4. *Describe the health care practices of early civilizations.*

5. *Discuss the three major historic images of the nurse.*

6. *Describe how each of these historic images has influenced the development of nursing as a profession.*

7. *Explain the significance of the "Dark Ages of Nursing" to the development of the nursing profession.*

8. *Discuss the contribution of Florence Nightingale to the development of nursing as a profession.*

9. *List some early hospitals established in the Americas.*

10. *Describe the early development of nursing schools in the United States.*

1

11. *Discuss factors that have affected the image of nursing today.*

12. *Identify at least three studies about nursing and explain why each is important.*

Key Terms

body of specialized
   knowledge
code of ethics
Dark Ages of Nursing
Florence Nightingale
formal characteristics
image
folk image
religious image

servant image
institutions of higher
   education
medicine
nursing
occupation
profession
professional
traditions

Situations to Foster Critical Thinking

1. Develop a definition of nursing that reflects your beliefs about the role and responsibilities of today's nurse. Compare and contrast your definition with the definitions of three major nursing theorists. Defend concepts that you have included that differ from those of each theorist. (Objective 2)

2. You are asked to do a presentation for a group of prenursing students on nursing as a profession. Using the characteristics typically associated with professions, what factors will you emphasize? Which factors will you omit? Why did you make those choices? Are there additional factors that you believe should be considered? Provide a rationale for all of your answers. (Objective 3)

3. Of the three historical images of nursing discussed in your text, which do you believe had the strongest impact on nursing as a profession? Why do you believe this to be true? Do you believe this had a negative or positive impact? If it had been possible, how would you have changed the situation? (Objective 6)

4. If you were able to sit down and have a cup of coffee with Florence Nightingale, what would you want to ask her about nursing during the time she was alive? What would you want to share with her about nursing education today? How would you describe the role of the nurse in today's world for her? (Objectives 6, 8, 11)

5. Identify at least three issues that you believe need to be studied with regard to nursing as it is currently being practiced. Provide a rationale

for these studies? How will nursing benefit? Who should do the studies? What might be some of the outcomes? What might be the impact on health care reform? (Objectives 11, 12)

6. Take a position on one of the traditions in nursing? Develop a rationale for its continuance or demise? What will be the effect of either? (Objective 11)

7. Of the five major categories of issues identified by the National Commission for the Study of Nursing and Nursing Education, which do you see as most critical? Provide a rationale for your answer. (Objective 12)

Discussion/Essay Questions

1. What factors have hampered the profession in defining nursing? (Objective 1)

2. How would you define nursing? (Objective 2)

3. Which nursing theory does your definition of nursing most closely parallel and who was its author? (Objective 2)

4. How does nursing differ from medicine? (Objective 2)

5. Define the terms *profession* and *professional*. (Objective 3)

6. Identify five generally accepted characteristics of a profession. For each characteristic, discuss the extent to which you think nursing meets this standard. (Objective 3)

7. What is meant by the term *body of specialized knowledge*? (Objective 3)

8. Which of the criteria that an occupation must meet to be a profession do some persons believe nursing fails to meet? (Objective 3)

9. Describe the approach to medicine seen in five early cultures, identifying the unique practices of each culture. (Objective 4)

10. Identify the three historical images of nursing and discuss why each existed. (Objective 5)

11. How has nursing been influenced by early religious movements? (Objective 6)

12. How has nursing been influenced by military activities? (Objective 6)

13. To what extent has nursing been affected by the women's movement? (Objective 6)

14. What events led to the "Dark Ages" in nursing? (Objective 7)

15. Who was Sairey Gamp? (Objective 7)

16. Discuss the contributions Florence Nightingale made to the nursing profession. (Objective 8)

17. Identify at least four basic principles that Florence Nightingale believed were essential for a sound nursing program. (Objective 8)

18. Where were the first hospitals founded in the United States? (Objective 9)

19. Discuss the development of early hospitals and explain why they were located where they were. (Objective 9)

20. Where and when was the first nursing school established in the United States? (Objective 10)

21. What were the characteristics of early nursing schools? (Objective 10)

22. Discuss the image of nursing today. (Objective 11)

23. Of the many media that influence nursing's image, which offer the most accurate portrayal? Why? (Objective 11)

24. Why are nurses concerned about the image of nursing? (Objective 11)

25. What was the thrust of early studies of nursing and why was it important at the time? (Objective 12)

26. What was the focus of nursing studies conducted during the middle of the 20th century and why were they completed? (Objective 12)

27. Discuss the focus of the study conducted by the National Commission for the Study of Nursing and Nursing Education published under the title *From Abstract to Action.* (Objective 12)

28. Do you believe that nursing as a profession lacks cohesiveness? Why? (Objectives 11, 12)

29. Compare and contrast the major findings of the Institute of Medicine study with the nursing situation today. (Objective 12)

30. Identify the reasons that you believe nursing pinning ceremonies should be continued or discontinued? (Objective 11)

Fill-In-The-Blank

1. In general, medicine is concerned with the _____ and _____ of disease. (Objective 1)

2. One of the factors significantly affecting the definition of nursing and the role of the nurse is _____ advances. (Objective 1)

3. The nurse theorist who developed a definition of nursing for the International Council of Nurses was _____. (Objective 2)

4. Two professional groups that have developed definitions of nursing are the _____ and the _____. (Objective 2)

5. Today, by far the majority of nursing programs preparing registered nurses are located in _____. (Objective 3)

6. The general standard for professional behavior of nurses in the United States is the American Nurses Association _____ _____. (Objective 3)

7. The oldest medical records so far discovered and deciphered came from _____. (Objective 4)

8. The early Hebrew culture is credited with having an organized method of _____. (Objective 4)

9. The Chinese believed in a philosophy of _____ and _____, two forces that are considered to contrast with, and be complimentary to, one another. (Objective 4)

10. Hippocrates, the Father of Medicine, came from the _____ culture. (Objective 4)

11. The three images of nursing identified by Uprichard are the _____ image, the _____ image, and the _____ image. (Objective 5)

12. Individuals who contributed significantly to the history of nursing include the _____ in the Eastern churches. (Objective 6)

13. Three Roman "matrons" who are remembered in the history of nursing are _____, _____, and _____. (Objective 6)

14. One of the outcomes of the Reformation that significantly affected nursing was a _____ _____. (Objective 7)

15. The "Dark Ages" in nursing were precipitated by the _____ _____. (Objective 7)

16. The individual who reformed the care of British soldiers wounded in the Crimean War was _____ _____. (Objective 8)

17. The first hospital founded in the United States was the _____. (Objective 9)

18. The American Red Cross was founded by _____ _____. (Objective 10)

19. The first nursing program was established at the _____ _____ _____ in 1872. (Objective 10)

20. The media that most accurately reflect the image of the nurse are _____ and _____. (Objective 11)

21. _____ was well known for her concern for the mentally ill as well as her appointment as superintendent of women nurses for the Union Army. (Objective 11)

22. Three nurses who carried out nursing duties for the Union army while supporting antislavery activities for the blacks were _____, _____, and _____. (Objective 11)

23. The early studies of nursing focused on _____ _____. (Objective 12)

24. The Study of Nursing and Nursing Education in the United States is known as the _____ _____. (Objective 12)

25. A study of nursing that resulted in the development of associate degree programs was conducted by _____ _____. (Objective 12)

26. Responding to the increasing need for nurses, many of the studies of the early 1990s focused on _____ _____. (Objective 12)

27. Many nursing programs have continued the tradition of awarding a ___ _____ to graduates when they complete their program of study. (Objective 11)

28. Two areas of the acute care hospital in which uniforms might not be worn are the _____ unit and the _____ unit. (Objective 11)

29. The nursing cap would seem reasonably to have evolved out of the period of time when nursing was greatly influenced by _____. (Objectives 5, 11)

30. The Institute of Medicine study made _____ specific recommendations to Congress regarding nursing. (Objective 12)

True-False Questions

____ 1. Most nurses have been able to agree on a definition of nursing. (Objective 1)

____ 2. The fact that there are several educational routes to registered nursing has complicated the process of defining nursing. (Objective 1)

____ 3. Technological advances have affected the definition of nursing. (Objective 1)

____ 4. The fact that the majority of nurses are women has had little effect on the definition of nursing. (Objective 1)

____ 5. Some believe that nursing falls short of meeting the criterion that a profession has a "body of specialized knowledge." (Objective 2)

____ 6. Studies of nursing indicate that most individuals who get an education that prepares them for nursing remain with the profession. (Objective 3)

_____ 7. One of the earliest organizations for men in nursing was known as the Parabolani brotherhood. (Objective 4)

_____ 8. The Knights Hospitallers of St. John was one of the orders to evolve from the Civil War. (Objective 4)

_____ 9. Continuity in the history of nursing began with Christianity. (Objective 6)

_____ 10. The military nursing orders were eliminated by the Crusades. (Objective 6)

_____ 11. The Reformation led to the establishment of Catholic churches and hospitals throughout Europe. (Objective 7)

_____ 12. Florence Nightingale crusaded for and brought about great reform in nursing education. (Objective 8)

_____ 13. Florence Nightingale believed that an important aspect of nurses' work involved cleaning. (Objective 8)

_____ 14. The first hospital founded in the United States was started in Philadelphia in 1751. (Objective 9)

_____ 15. Benjamin Franklin fought hospital development in the United States. (Objective 9)

_____ 16. The first nursing programs in the United States were established on the west coast. (Objective 10)

_____ 17. The image of nursing reached a low point in the 1970s. (Objective 11)

_____ 18. In studying nurses on television, Kalisch and Kalisch found that nurses often had no substantive role in the television stories. (Objective 11)

_____ 19. Newspapers and news magazines tend to project the most accurate image of nursing today. (Objective 11)

_____ 20. The first recommendation of the Institute of Medicine study was that the federal government discontinue efforts to increase the supply of "generalist" nurses. (Objective 12)

Matching Questions

Match the numbered statements with the lettered names.

A. 1. Developed a definition of nursing (Objective 1)

2. Established the first monastery for women (Objective 8)

3. Was a nursing character in one of Dickens' novels (Objective 10)

4. Cared for soldiers in the Crimean War (Objective 10)

5. Served as superintendent of women nurses during the Civil War (Objective 6)

6. Conducted one of the early studies of nursing (Objective 12)

    ____ a. Sairey Gamp

    ____ b. Florence Nightingale

    ____ c. Dorothea Dix

    ____ d. M. Adelaide Nutting

    ____ e. Virginia Henderson

    ____ f. St. Marcella

B. 1. Recorded information about health practices in a sacred book called the Vedas

2. Established early schools for priest—physicians who healed either by knife, with herbs, or through exorcism

3. Believed that illness was a punishment for sin

4. Built exquisite temples that became places to obtain cures

5. Often borrowed medical practices from countries they conquered

6. Believed in a balance between the yang and the yin (all Objective 4)

    ____ a. Assyria

    ____ b. China

    ____ c. Greece

    ____ d. India

    ____ e. Persia

    ____ f. The Romans

Multiple-Choice Questions

_____ 1. Which of the following is one reason why we have had difficulty defining nursing?

    a. The advancing technology in the health fields has changed the role of the nurse.

    b. Nurses have been unwilling to accept changing roles.

    c. The public is not responsive to defining nursing.

    d. Hospital administrations block efforts to define nursing.

    (Objective 1)

_____ 2. The term _registered nurse_ (RN) represents

    a. a legal title.

    b. a descriptive title.

    c. a college degree.

    d. none of the above.

    (Objective 1)

_____ 3. "A Social Policy Statement" that provided a definition of nursing was developed by

    a. the National League for Nursing.

    b. the American Nurses Association.

    c. the National Council of State Boards of Nursing.

    d. the National Student Nurse Association.

    (Objective 2)

_____ 4. The single most important part of any Nurse Practice Act is

    a. establishing a rate of pay for registered nurses.

    b. defining incompetent practice.

    c. establishing a legal definition of nursing practice.

    d. establishing the roles of the various members of the board.

    (Objective 2)

_____ 5. Which one of the following would most authors include as a characteristic of a profession?

    a.   A profession licenses all its practitioners.

    b.   A profession should develop and enforce its own code of ethics.

    c.   A profession mandates continuing education for continued practice.

    d.   A profession limits the number of persons who can enter the profession.

    (Objective 3)

_____ 6. The culture that developed elaborate materia medica was the ancient

    a.   Babylonians.

    b.   Brahmans.

    c.   Chinese.

    d.   Persians.

_____ 7. The first hospitals, established about 50 AD to 800 AD, usually were located

    a.   near battlefields.

    b.   in the homes of private citizens.

    c.   near monasteries.

    d.   in the center of large cities.

    (Objective 4)

_____ 8. The Mosaic Code, which represented an organized method of disease prevention, was developed by which of the following early cultures?

    a.   Ancient Chinese

    b.   Hebrews

    c.   Early Hindus

    d.   Greeks

    (Objective 4)

_____ 9. One of the three historical images of the nurse identified by Uprichard is that of

    a.   handmaiden.

    b.   battle-axe.

    c.   angel of mercy.

    d.   servant.

(Objective 5)

_____ 10. The early deaconesses sometimes are identified as the early counterparts of which branch of nursing today?

    a.   Community health nurses

    b.   Epidemiologists (disease control nurses)

    c.   Nurse anesthetists

    d.   Critical care nurses

(Objective 6)

_____ 11. One of the early Roman matrons who significantly contributed to nursing was

    a.   Christina.

    b.   St. Maria.

    c.   Marcella.

    d.   Anastasia.

(Objective 6)

_____ 12. Historically, the development of nursing as a profession was influenced by military factors. It also was significantly influenced by

    a.   economic situations.

    b.   environmental conditions.

    c.   religious movements.

    d.   none of the above.

(Objective 6)

_____ 13. The <u>Order of Widows</u> was a title used by an early nursing group to designate
   a.   marital status.
   b.   respect for age.
   c.   religious affiliation.
   d.   commitment to purity of life.
   (Objective 6)

_____ 14. The effects of the Reformation during the 16th century created which of the following in nursing?
   a.   The Renaissance
   b.   The birth of modern nursing
   c.   The "Dark Ages" in nursing
   d.   The development of nursing schools
   (Objective 7)

_____ 15. The Reformation affected nursing in that it
   a.   changed the role of the Pope.
   b.   encouraged people to be free thinkers.
   c.   enhanced the image of nursing at that time.
   d.   changed the role of women at that time.
   (Objective 7)

_____ 16. Florence Nightingale's birthday is celebrated each year by our observance of
   a.   National Hospital Week.
   b.   Nurse Education Week.
   c.   National Public Health Week.
   d.   Veterans' Day.
   (Objective 8)

_____ 17. One of Florence Nightingale's major contributions to nursing was
   a.   bringing nurses to the war front.
   b.   writing nurses' notes.
   c.   establishing standards for nursing schools.
   d.   establishing the profession as separate from medicine.
   (Objective 8)

____ 18. The first person to begin advancing nursing as a profession was
   a.   Florence Nightingale.
   b.   Virginia Henderson.
   c.   Sairey Gamp.
   d.   Dorothea Dix.
   (Objective 8)

____ 19. The first hospital founded in the United States was located in the
city of
   a.   Jamestown.
   b.   New York.
   c.   Philadelphia.
   d.   Washington, DC.
   (Objective 9)

____ 20. The individual credited with being instrumental in establishing the
first hospital in the United States was
   a.   Benjamin Franklin.
   b.   John Henry.
   c.   Thomas Jefferson.
   d.   George Washington.

____ 21. Early nursing schools in the United States
   a.   were founded in colleges and universities.
   b.   had fairly standard curricula.
   c.   were well financed.
   d.   were fashioned after the Nightingale model.
   (Objective 10)

____ 22. The person appointed as superintendent of women nurses for the
Union Army during the Civil War was
   a.   Mildred Montag.
   b.   Florence Nightingale.
   c.   Dorothea Dix.
   d.   Clara Barton.
   (Objective 11)

___ 23. Walt Whitman wrote about nursing. Another author who did so was
    a.   Louisa May Alcott.
    b.   Joseph Wamburg.
    c.   Jack London.
    d.   Ayn Rand.
    (Objective 11)

___ 24. During the late 1970s and the early 1980s, a great deal of time and energy was invested in
    a.   the development of associate degree programs.
    b.   establishing mandatory licensure in all states.
    c.   developing a uniform disciplinary code.
    d.   studying the image of nursing.
    (Objective 11)

___ 25. In novels, most nurses have been portrayed as
    a.   married, female, and mothers.
    b.   male, married, and under 35.
    c.   single, female, and under 35.
    d.   over 35, male or female, and married.
    (Objective 11)

___ 26. Nurses have found that one effective method of responding to television advertisements or programs that portray nurses and nursing in a negative light is to
    a.   boycott purchase of the items advertised.
    b.   write to their congressman.
    c.   ignore the reference to nursing.
    d.   write to the consumer affairs department.
    (Objective 11)

___ 27. The earliest studies of nursing were concerned with
    a.   nursing education.
    b.   nursing practice.
    c.   nursing as a profession.
    d.   the funding of nursing research.
    (Objective 12)

_____ 28. The study entitled "Twenty Thousand Nurses Tell Their Story" provided information regarding

    a.   nursing salaries.

    b.   nursing curricula.

    c.   nurses themselves.

    d.   future nursing needs.

(Objective 12)

_____ 29. The Institute of Medicine study recommended that

    a.   more money be allocated to nursing education.

    b.   the federal government discontinue efforts to increase the supply of "generalist nurses."

    c.   nurses be required to have a baccalaureate degree to practice registered nursing.

    d.   all nursing programs be run in conjunction with a medical school.

(Objective 12)

_____ 30. The study entitled _Nursing for the Future_ was conducted by

    a.   Jerome Lysaught.

    b.   William Flexner.

    c.   Esther Lucille Brown.

    d.   Mildred Montag.

(Objective 12)

2 | Educational Preparation for Nursing

Purpose

Chapter 2 discusses the various forms and types of nursing education in the United States. Starting with the education of the nursing assistant and progressing through the doctoral program that prepares assistant graduates for registered nurse licensure, the various educational programs are described, and a historical review is provided. Also outlined are nontraditional approaches to nursing education and articulated programs. The chapter concludes with a discussion of continuing education and the issue of making continuing education for licensure mandatory.

Objectives

1. Describe the educational preparation and role of the nursing assistant.

2. Describe the educational preparation and role of the licensed practical nurse.

3. Discuss the educational preparation provided by a hospital-based diploma program of nursing.

4. Discuss the educational preparation provided by a baccalaureate degree program of nursing.

5. Discuss the educational preparation provided by an associate degree program of nursing.

6. Identify the purposes of other forms of nursing education: the external degree, registered nurse baccalaureate programs, master's preparation, doctoral studies, and nondegree programs.

7. Discuss the concept of articulated programs.

8. Define the continuing education unit and discuss its purpose.

9. Compare and contrast the major points supporting mandatory continuing education and the major points supporting voluntary continuing education.

Key Terms

articulation
associate degree
baccalaureate
diploma
doctorate
external degree
internship

mandatory continuing
  education
nursing assistant
practical (vocational)
registered nurse
  baccalaureate
voluntary continuing
  education

Situations to Foster Critical Thinking

1. Some believe that the number of educational routes to preparation as a registered nurse has resulted in public confusion and may detract from nursing's standing as a profession. Analyze your thoughts regarding this issue and develop a rationale for your position. How do you see nursing hampered by the number of ways one can prepare for licensure? What do you see as the strengths? Which are stronger? (Objectives 1-6)

2. Your friend, Betsy McClintock, wants to become a registered nurse. Because you have almost completed your program, she seeks your advice about whether to enter an associate degree or a baccalaureate degree program. In responding to her what questions would you ask? What would you tell her about each program? What would you identify as the strengths of each? Where would you send her for additional information?

3. Alice Wright is a certified nursing assistant who has worked on our nursing team at Valley Memorial Hospital. She is considering continuing her education as a practical or registered nurse and asks you about the difference between the two programs, both of which are available to her at the local community college. How would you describe the differences in scope of practice? Responsibility? Educational preparation? Job opportunities? Salary? (Objectives 2, 5, 7)

4. You have just accepted a position in a small hospital in a rural community in a state in which continuing education is not mandatory. There are no colleges or universities within 300 miles. Develop a plan for your own continuing education? What opportunities will be available to you? How will you pursue these? How can you be assured your practice will remain current? (Objectives 8, 9)

Discussion/Essay Questions

1. Do you think it is necessary to legislate educational preparation for nursing assistants? Why? (Objective 1)

2. What are the limitations of the activities nursing assistants can do for patients? (Objective 1)

3. What is the length of study for most nursing assistant programs? (Objective 1)

4. Discuss the development of educational programs that prepare practical nurses. (Objective 2)

5. Why was it logical to locate the first practical nurse program in a YWCA? (Objective 2)

6. Where are practical nursing programs located today? (Objective 2)

7. What is the official organization for practical nurses and when was it founded? (Objective 2)

8. Describe the nature and length of practical nurse programs. (Objective 2)

9. Discuss the scope of practice of the practical nurse. (Objective 2)

10. How does the practice of the practical nurse differ from that of a registered nurse? (Objectives 2-5)

11. Describe the educational program of the early "training schools" that were located in hospitals. (Objective 3)

12. Describe the characteristics of the students who enrolled in the early training schools. (Objectives 3)

13. Explain why there has been a decline in the number of diploma schools throughout the United States. (Objective 3)

14. Discuss the characteristics of the educational program offered by hospital-based diploma programs today. (Objective 3)

15. When and where was the first program leading to a baccalaureate degree in nursing founded? (Objective 4)

16. Discuss the characteristics of baccalaureate nursing education. (Objective 4)

17. What are the role and the scope of practice of a graduate of a baccalaureate degree nursing program? (Objective 4)

18. When and by whom were the first associate degree nursing programs founded? (Objective 5)

19. Why did the concept of associate degree nursing education grow so rapidly? (Objective 5)

20. Describe the characteristics of the students who enter associate degree nursing programs. (Objective 5)

21. Discuss the role and scope of practice of the graduate of an associate degree program. (Objective 5)

22. What are some of the issues that have resulted from the success of the associate degree programs in nursing? (Objective 5)

23. List at least four similarities among the programs that prepare graduates to write the licensing examination for registered nursing. (Objectives 3-5)

24. Describe the concept of the external degree. (Objective 6)

25. How does the New York Regents External Degree program in nursing differ from traditional programs? (Objective 6)

26. Describe the programs that lead to a master's degree in nursing and prepare the graduate for licensure. (Objectives 6, 7)

27. What is the purpose of RNB programs in nursing? (0bjectives 6, 7)

28. Identify at least three areas of concern with regard to RNB education. (Objective 6)

29. Describe the nature of a master's in nursing program. (Objective 6)

30. What roles are being filled in the health care delivery system by persons with master's preparation in nursing? (Objective 6)

31. Briefly discuss doctoral preparation in nursing. (Objective 6)

32. Why have internship programs for new graduates enjoyed such wide popularity? (Objective 6)

33. Describe what a continuing education unit is and explain the purpose of such units. (Objective 8)

34. Discuss the major arguments advanced in support of mandatory continuing education in nursing and the major arguments advanced in support of making such education voluntary. (Objective 9)

Fill-In-The-Blank Questions

1. Federal legislation that regulates the education and certification of nurse aides is called the _____. (Objective 1)

2. The certified nursing assistant (CNA) functions under the direction of _____ or the _____. (Objective 1)

3. The state agency bearing the responsibility for regarding or certifying nursing assistants _____. (Objective 1)

4. It is a popular belief that the first programs for practical nurses were initiated through the _____ in New York. (Objective 2)

5. In general, the curriculum for practical nursing lasts _____ month(s) to _____ year(s). (Objective 2)

6. Licensed practical nurses are titled licensed _____ nurses in Texas and California. (Objective 2)

7. Practical nurse education gained a firm position in the decade of the __ _____. (Objective 2)

8. The majority of programs preparing practical nurses are located in _____ _____ _____. (Objective 2)

9. The three avenues preparing men and women for registered nursing are _____ programs, _____ programs, and _____ _____ programs. (Objectives 3-5)

10. The majority of registered nurses practicing today gained their basic nursing education in _____ _____ programs. (Objective 3)

11. When certain learning experiences were not available in the hospital offering the diploma program, students were sent on _____ to another facility. (Objective 3)

12. One of the strengths of the diploma programs, as seen by employers, was that the new graduate could _____ __.(Objective 3)

13. A major factor that has resulted in the decrease in the number of diploma programs has been the _____. (Objective 3)

14. The first program in nursing leading to a baccalaureate degree was located at _____. (Objective 4)

15. Baccalaureate nursing education is based on a foundation of _____ __. (Objective 4)

16. Baccalaureate nursing education programs are located in _____ and _____ . (Objective 4)

17. The type of nursing program that places strong emphasis on supervision and leadership techniques is the _____ _____. (Objective 4)

18. The first associate degree programs were started in the year _____. (Objective 5)

19. The architect of the concept of associate degree education is _____. (Objective 5)

20. The majority of associate degree nursing programs are located in _____ _____. (Objective 5)

21. Additional programs that lead to a baccalaureate degree in nursing are available to graduates of associate degree and diploma programs and are referred to as _____.(Objective 6)

22. Specialization in nursing occurs at the _____ level. (Objective 6)

23. Programs run by hospitals that are intended to ease the transition from the role of student to that of staff by providing an opportunity to increase clinical skills and knowledge are known as _____. (Objective 6)

24. Planned learning experiences developed for the new graduate and operated by the hospital may be called _____, _____, or _____. (Objective 6)

25. Nondegree programs would include those specialized programs that have been developed to _____ . (Objective 6)

26. A program that provides direct movement between a lower-level and a higher-level program in nursing is referred to as a (an) _____ program. (Objective 7)

27. Articulated programs in nursing are also sometimes referred to as _____ programs. (Objective 7)

28. Continuing education programs are frequently presented in association with _____. (Objective 8)

29. A "planned learning experience beyond a basic nursing education program" is called _____. (Objective 8)

30. Continuing education may be either _____ or _____, depending on a particular state's laws. (Objective 8)

True-False Questions

_____ 1. The preparation of the nursing assistant is limited to on-the-job training. (Objective 1)

_____ 2. The Nurse Aide Competency Evaluation Programs (NACEP) can be used as a guide by programs registering or certifying nursing aides. (Objective 1)

_____ 3. Each state identifies the skills that may be performed by the nursing assistant. (Objective 1)

_____ 4. All states require that the nursing assistant participate in continuing education. (Objective 1)

_____ 5. The practical nurse is no newcomer to the health care delivery system. (Objective 2)

_____ 6. Graduates of diploma programs write the National Council Licensing Examination for practical nursing. (Objective 2)

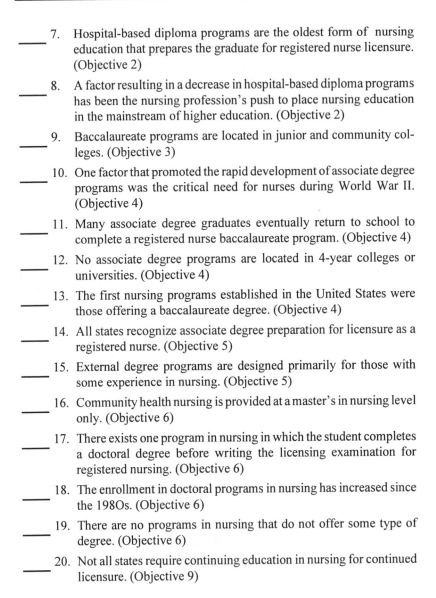

_____ 7. Hospital-based diploma programs are the oldest form of nursing education that prepares the graduate for registered nurse licensure. (Objective 2)

_____ 8. A factor resulting in a decrease in hospital-based diploma programs has been the nursing profession's push to place nursing education in the mainstream of higher education. (Objective 2)

_____ 9. Baccalaureate programs are located in junior and community colleges. (Objective 3)

_____ 10. One factor that promoted the rapid development of associate degree programs was the critical need for nurses during World War II. (Objective 4)

_____ 11. Many associate degree graduates eventually return to school to complete a registered nurse baccalaureate program. (Objective 4)

_____ 12. No associate degree programs are located in 4-year colleges or universities. (Objective 4)

_____ 13. The first nursing programs established in the United States were those offering a baccalaureate degree. (Objective 4)

_____ 14. All states recognize associate degree preparation for licensure as a registered nurse. (Objective 5)

_____ 15. External degree programs are designed primarily for those with some experience in nursing. (Objective 5)

_____ 16. Community health nursing is provided at a master's in nursing level only. (Objective 6)

_____ 17. There exists one program in nursing in which the student completes a doctoral degree before writing the licensing examination for registered nursing. (Objective 6)

_____ 18. The enrollment in doctoral programs in nursing has increased since the 1980s. (Objective 6)

_____ 19. There are no programs in nursing that do not offer some type of degree. (Objective 6)

_____ 20. Not all states require continuing education in nursing for continued licensure. (Objective 9)

Matching Questions

Match the numbered terms with the lettered statements.

A. 1. Regents external degree (Objective 5)

2. Master's degree in nursing (Objective 6)

3. Baccalaureate degree in nursing (Objective 3)

    4. Associate degree nursing programs (Objective 4)

    5. Hospital-based diploma education (Objective 2)

    6. Practical nursing education (Objective 1)

        ____ a. Early programs were located in the YWCA.

        ____ b. The first programs were started in 1952.

        ____ c. The first program was started at the University of Minnesota.

        ____ d. The program is built on the concept of assessment of knowledge.

        ____ e. Most of today's practicing nurses received their basic education from this type of program.

        ____ f. This program provides for specialization in nursing.

B. 1. Doctoral programs in nursing (Objective 6)

    2. Associate degree programs (Objective 4)

    3. Diploma programs (Objective 2)

    4. Baccalaureate degree programs (Objective 3)

    5. Practical nurse programs (Objective 1)

        ____ a. Programs are located primarily in vocational-technical institutes or community colleges.

        ____ b. Programs are located primarily in community college settings.

        ____ c. Programs are located in senior colleges and universities.

        ____ d. Programs are located in hospitals.

        ____ e. Programs are located in multiuniversity settings.

Multiple-Choice Questions

____ 1. What are the minimum number of hours of theory required in the preparation of a nursing assistant?

      a. 25 hours

      b. 50 hours

      c. 75 hours

      d. 100 hours

    (Objective 1)

_____ 2. It is believed that the first programs to offer formal preparation for practical nursing began in
  a. junior colleges.
  b. state universities
  c. the YWCA
  d. the churches.
  (Objective 2)

_____ 3. The first accrediting service for practical nursing programs was established by
  a. the American Nurses Association.
  b. the National League for Nursing.
  c. the National Federation of Licensed Practical Nurses.
  d. the Association of Practical Nurse Education and Service.
  (Objective 2)

_____ 4. The practical nurse is known as a vocational nurse in the states of
  a. California and Texas.
  b. Montana and Utah.
  c. North Carolina and South Carolina.
  d. New York and New Jersey.
  (Objective 2)

_____ 5. What is the period of study of most practical nurse programs?
  a. 6 months
  b. 9 months to 1 year
  c. 18 months
  d. 24 months
  (Objective 2)

____ 6. The type of nursing programs that might be located in a high school, trade or technical school, hospital, junior or community college, university, or independent agency is most likely to be a (an)

  a. nurse aide program or practical nurse program.

  b. associate degree program.

  c. baccalaureate degree program.

  d. master's degree program.

  (Objectives 1, 2)

____ 7. The earliest schools of nursing were located in

  a. community colleges.

  b. hospitals.

  c. senior colleges and universities.

  d. vocational-technical institutes.

  (Objective 3)

____ 8. The majority of registered nurses practicing today gained their basic nursing education in

  a. associate degree programs.

  b. articulated programs.

  c. baccalaureate programs.

  d. diploma programs.

  (Objective 3)

____ 9. Diploma programs are located in

  a. community colleges.

  b. technical-vocational institutes.

  c. hospitals.

  d. universities.

  (Objectives 3)

____ 10. How long is the traditional diploma program?

  a. 1 year

  b. 2 years

  c. 3 years

  d. 4 years

  (Objective 3)

_____ 11. The person recognized as being the first nurse graduate in the United States is
   a.   Carrie Lenburgh.
   b.   Isabelle Hampton Robb.
   c.   Philomena Witherstone.
   d.   Linda Richards.
   (Objective 3)

_____ 12. The first baccalaureate nursing program was started at the University of Minnesota in
   a.   1853.
   b.   1875.
   c.   1909.
   d.   1922.
   (Objective 4)

_____ 13. Baccalaureate nursing programs are located in
   a.   senior colleges and universities.
   b.   community colleges.
   c.   hospitals.
   d.   vocational-technical institutes.
   (Objective 4)

_____ 14. The type of nursing program that provides experience in community nursing is the
   a.   practical nurse program.
   b.   diploma program.
   c.   associate degree program.
   d.   baccalaureate program.
   (Objective 4)

_____ 15. The type of nursing education program founded on the premise that the health care delivery system could incorporate a nursing technician was

    a.   the certified aide program.

    b.   the licenced practical nurse program.

    c.   the hospital-based diploma program.

    d.   the associate degree program.

    (Objective 5)

_____ 16. Associate degree nursing programs are usually located in

    a.   senior colleges and universities.

    b.   community colleges.

    c.   hospitals.

    d.   vocational-technical institutes.

    (Objective 5)

_____ 17. The newest form of nursing education is the associate degree program. The architect for these programs is

    a.   Ester Lucille Brown.

    b.   Mildred Montag.

    c.   Adelaide Nutting.

    d.   Virginia Henderson.

    (Objective 5)

_____ 18. Graduates of associate degree programs are prepared to

    a.   work in public health situations.

    b.   relieve the head nurse.

    c.   teach continuing education courses to licensed practical nurses.

    d.   work as staff nurses on a medical/surgical unit.

    (Objective 5)

_____ 19. Which of the following would be the most appropriate position for a new graduate from an associate degree program?

   a. School nurse

   b. Staff nurse on a medical/surgical unit of an acute care facility

   c. Change nurse on the 3-to-11 shift in a long-term care facility

   d. Instructor in a licensed practical nurse program

   (Objective 5)

_____ 20. The type of program in which there are no prescribed methods of learning and in which learning is assessed through highly standardized and validated examinations is known as

   a. an open curriculum.

   b. self-paced learning.

   c. an external degree program.

   d. an articulated program.

   (Objective 6)

_____ 21. Specialization in nursing occurs at what level of education?

   a. Associate degree

   b. Baccalaureate degree

   c. Master's degree

   d. Doctoral degree

   (Objective 6)

_____ 22. Programs that provide baccalaureate education to registered nurses are known as

   a. basic programs.

   b. external degree programs.

   c. ladder programs.

   d. RNB programs.

   (Objective 6)

____ 23. The term RNB is used to refer to
   a.   two-year generic programs.
   b.   four-year generic programs.
   c.   programs that provide baccalaureate education to registered nurses.
   d.   programs that require completion of a nurse aide program before practical nursing and of practical nursing before associate degree nursing.
   (Objective 6)

____ 24. One of the major problems associated with RNB programs relates to
   a.   the accreditation of the program.
   b.   the large number of applicants.
   c.   the evaluation of previous learning.
   d.   the qualifications of the faculty.
   (Objective 6)

____ 25. The critical need for nurses to fulfill the expanded role of the nurse has resulted in the increase of which type of program?
   a.   Associate degree
   b.   Baccalaureate degree
   c.   Master's degree
   d.   Doctoral degree
   (Objective 6)

____ 26. Which of the following statements is true of doctoral programs in nursing?
   a.   Doctorates can be earned only in allied areas such as anthropology or education.
   b.   Doctorates in nursing are increasing.
   c.   Doctorates in nursing are decreasing.
   d.   Doctorates in nursing are required for all leadership positions.
   (Objective 8)

_____ 27. Programs that allow an individual to move smoothly from one level of nursing education to the next with minimal loss of earned credit are known as

    a. articulated programs.

    b. self-paced programs.

    c. external degree programs.

    d. RNB programs.

(Objective 7)

_____ 28. Articulated programs may also be known as

    a. two-on-two programs.

    b. external degree programs.

    c. continuing education programs.

    d. internships.

(Objective 7)

_____ 29. Which of the following is a requirement of all registered nurses in the United States?

    a. Take continuing education courses

    b. Pass institutional credentialing criteria

    c. Have a degree from an accredited college

    d. Pass the National Council Licensing Examination for Registered Nursing

(Objectives 2-4, 8, 9)

_____ 30. Which of the following statements is true?

    a. All states but one have mandatory continuing education requirements.

    b. Mandatory continuing education affects licensure.

    c. No states currently have mandatory continuing education requirements.

    d. Mandatory continuing education is an issue of declining interest in nursing.

(Objective 9)

3 | Perspectives on Nursing Education

Purpose

Chapter 3 discusses nursing education from a variety of perspectives. It outlines factors that have resulted in changes in nursing education, including the development of accreditation standards, the licensing examination, the changing role of the nurse, and some of the studies and reports that have focused on nursing. The activities that led up to the development of the American Nurses Association (ANA) position paper are discussed, as well as the positions taken by other organizations. Problems encountered in implementing the position paper are outlined, with specific attention paid to the issues surrounding titling and the grandfather clause. The concept of differentiated practice is examined along with a discussion of competency statements. A discussion of the impact of federal funding for nursing education and a brief review of the major nursing theorists conclude the chapter.

Objectives

1. *Discuss the impact of the Brown report.*

2. *Explain factors that prompted improvements in nursing education in the 1950s and 1960s.*

3. *Discuss the development and effect of the ANA position paper on nursing education and on nursing organizations.*

4. *Outline the arguments against the ANA position on entry from the viewpoint of associate degree and hospital-based schools.*

5. *Explain what is meant by a grandfather clause and the effect of such a clause on responses to proposed changes in nursing licensure.*

6. *Analyze the problems created for nursing mobility by changes in individual state licensure laws.*

7. *Discuss the concept of differentiated practice and provide a rationale for its development.*

8. *Explain how the nursing shortage, computers in health care, and changes to community-based practice have had an impact on nursing education.*

31

9. *Discuss the impact of reduced federal funding on nursing education.*

10. *Explain why nursing theories are important to the profession.*

11. *Identify one theory that you believe describes nursing as it should be practiced and give your rationale for selecting this theory.*

Key Terms

advanced practice	entry into practice
accreditation	grandfather clause
associate degree	hospital-based program
baccalaureate degree	interstate endorsement
community based	position paper
competencies	scope of practice
differentiated practice	theorists/theory
education mobility	titling

Situations to Foster Critical Thinking

1. If you were able to develop a plan for nursing education that would be adopted by the profession, what would that plan include? What testing mechanism would you put in place? How would you manage interstate endorsement? (Objectives 1-4, 6)

2. Do you believe that grandfather clauses should be continued? Make a case for your answer. If you support grandfather clauses as they exist, give the reasons you believe some persons should unconditionally be allowed to continue to practice under old rules or regulations. If you believe grandfathering should be conditional, defend your position. How would you determine how long the conditional time should be? What would you recommend if the conditions were not met? (Objective 5)

3. Do you believe that hospitals should incorporate differentiated practice into their staffing patterns? Provide the rationale for your answer. Would you tie salary to the type of educational preparation for registered nurses? Why or why not? (Objective 7)

4. Do you believe that the federal government should continue to allocate money for nursing education? Why? If you believe they should, give reasons that you believe nursing should be given the funds when many other professions are not? If you believe they should not, what other mechanisms might be available to assist with the funding of nursing education? (Objective 9)

5.   Select one of the nursing theories discussed in the text. Outline how it explains nursing as you believe it should be practiced. Why did you select that theory? Why do you think that theory is important to nursing? What weaknesses, if any, do you see in the theory? (Objectives 10, 11)

Discussion/Essay Questions

1.   Discuss one of the major recommendations of the Brown report and identify its significance to nursing as a profession. (Objective 1)

2.   Discuss activities that occurred in the 1950s and resulted in changes in nursing. (Objective 2)

3.   How did the development of uniform licensing affect nursing education? (Objective 2)

4.   Do you believe that nursing schools should meet national standards (i.e., be accredited)? Why? (Objective 2)

5.   Outline the events in nursing that led to the development of the ANA's first position paper on nursing education. (Objective 3)

6.   What were the major assumptions on which the ANA position paper was based? (Objective 3)

7.   What were the four positions outlined in the ANA position paper? (Objective 3)

8.   Why do you believe the ANA position paper has not been implemented? (Objectives 3, 4)

9.   In general, what has been the response of other organizations to the ANA position paper? (Objective 4)

10.   What has been the response of the various states to the ANA position paper? (Objective 4)

11.   Discuss the position of the North Dakota Board of Nursing. (Objective 4)

12.   What kinds of concerns surrounded the titling issue? (Objective 4)

13.   What is meant by scope of practice and how is it accepted by the entry-into-practice issue? (Objective 4)

14.   What is the grandfather clause and what is its purpose? (Objective 5)

15.   What is meant by interstate endorsement? (Objective 6)

16.   How might the entry issue affect interstate endorsement? (Objective 6)

17.   Discuss the concept of the grandfather clause and the reasons why it is necessary when some laws are changed. (Objective 5)

18.   Discuss the problems associated with defining the competencies of graduates of the various programs. (Objective 7)

19. Discuss the concept of differentiated practice and explain how, if implemented, it might change nursing education in the future. (Objective 7)

20. What are the results of having so many variously prepared health care providers in nursing? (Objective 7)

21. What changes might one anticipate in nursing education in the future and what would be the impetus for these changes? (Objective 8)

22. Describe how nursing benefited from federal funding in the past. (Objective 9)

23. How will nursing programs suffer from the loss of federal dollars invested in nursing education? (Objective 9)

24. If federal funding for nursing education is lost, what other ways might nursing education be supported? (Objective 9)

25. What is meant by a theory of nursing? (Objective 10)

26. Why has the development of nursing theories flourished in the nursing profession? (Objective 10)

27. Identify some of the nursing theorists who have developed nursing theories that speak to the art and science of humanistic nursing. (Objective 11)

28. Identify some nursing theorists who have developed nursing theories that involve interpersonal relationships. (Objective 11)

29. Identify some nursing theorists who have developed systems theories. (Objective 11)

30. What role do you see nursing theories playing in the development of nursing as a profession? (Objective 11)

Fill-In-The-Blank Questions

1. A report on nursing prepared by Ester Lucille Brown was titled _____ _____. (Objective 1)

2. Four factors that affect the way nursing is practiced are _____, _____, _____, and _____ factors. (Objective 2)

3. The professional nursing group that is responsible for accrediting nursing programs is the _____. (Objective 2)

4. The first position taken by the ANA position paper states that the education for all who practice nursing should take place in _____. (Objective 3)

5. According to the ANA position paper, the minimum educational preparation to practice professional nursing should be a (an) _____. (Objective 3)

6. According to the ANA position paper, the minimum educational preparation to practice technical nursing should be a (an) _____. (Objective 3)

7. As of January 1987, a baccalaureate degree is required for registered nursing in the state of _____. (Objective 6)

8. The section of the Nurse Practice Act that outlines the activities a person with that license may perform is referred to as the _____. (Objective 4)

9. When a state licensure law is changed, a _____ clause has been a standard feature that allows persons to continue to practice their occupation after new qualifications have been enacted into law. (Objective 5)

10. Two of the major issues surrounding the ANA position paper involve _____ and _____. (Objective 5)

11. The process that allows a nurse who has written and passed the licensure examination in one state to move to another and obtain a license without retaking the examination is known as _____. (Objective 6)

12. Moving toward differentiated practice would require defining the _____ of graduates of the various types of nursing education programs. (Objective 7)

13. One of the changes that is occurring in nursing education is the inclusion of content related to operating _____. (Objective 8)

14. One of the approaches to the changes in nursing supply has been an increased emphasis on _____. (Objective 8)

15. A significant change in nursing practice is the trend toward _____ practice. (Objective 8)

16. The bill that has made federal money available to nursing programs is called the _____. (Objective 9)

17. The nursing theory developed by Sister Callista Roy is known as a (an) _____ theory. (Objective 11)

18. The nursing theory developed by Betty Neuman might be identified as _____ theory. (Objective 11)

19. The nursing theory known as the science of unitary man was developed by _____. (Objective 11)

20. Dorothy Orem's theory of nursing focuses on the concept of _____. (Objective 11)

21. The individual noted for her development of a definition of nursing is _____. (Objective 11)

22.   Theories that deal with interactions between and among individuals are known as _____ theories. (Objective 11)

True-False Questions

_____   1.   The Brown report emerged because of concern for the fact that young women were not choosing nursing as a profession. (Objective 1)

_____   2.   Changes in nursing practice have required nurses prepared with higher levels of education. (Objective 2)

_____   3.   The report of the Surgeon General's Consultant Group found that the supply of nurses was adequate. (Objective 2)

_____   4.   The Nurse Training Act of 1964 was an outgrowth of the Surgeon General's report. (Objective 2)

_____   5.   As early as the 1950s, the ANA was concerned about the education for professional nursing. (Objective 3)

_____   6.   The ANA position paper on nursing education was first published in 1982. (Objective 3)

_____   7.   The ANA position paper on nursing education advocates a master's degree in nursing for the practice of professional nursing. (Objective 3)

_____   8.   The ANA position paper on nursing education proposes that all educational preparation for nursing occur in institutions of higher education. (Objective 3)

_____   9.   The ANA position paper on nursing education advocates that the minimum educational preparation for technical nursing be an associate degree in nursing. (Objective 3)

_____   10.   The ANA position paper on nursing education is based on an assumption that the demand for services of nurses will decrease. (Objective 3)

_____   11.   The ANA believes that the education for those in the health professions must increase in depth and breadth as scientific knowledge expands. (Objective 3)

_____   12.   At their 1987 convention, the membership of the NLN supported the title "registered associate nurse" for the associate degree graduate. (Objective 4)

_____   13.   The state of North Dakota now requires a baccalaureate degree in nursing to allow graduates to write the licensure examination for registered nursing. (Objective 6)

_____ 14. Most nursing organizations are not supportive of the concept of requiring a baccalaureate degree for professional nursing practice. (Objective 4)

_____ 15. The National Council of State Boards of Nursing has taken a formal position of neutrality on changes in nursing education requirements for entry. (Objective 3)

_____ 16. The National Federation of Licensed Practical Nurses has supported the concept of increasing the 1-year program to 18 months. (Objective 3)

_____ 17. The National Federation of Licensed Practical Nurses supports the ANA position that all education for nurses should occur in institutions of higher education. (Objective 3)

_____ 18. The National Federation of Licensed Practical Nurses supports the use of the title "associate nurse" for the graduate of the practical nurse programs of the future. (Objective 3)

_____ 19. The majority of practical nurse programs are no longer located in vocational-technical institutes. (Objective 3)

_____ 20. The titles to be used by persons working at each level have not been identified by many states. (Objective 4)

_____ 21. The scope of practice is that section of the Nurse Practice Act that outlines the activities a person with that license may engage in legally. (Objective 4)

_____ 22. When a state licensure law is changed, the grandfather clause allows persons to continue to practice their profession after new qualifications they might not have met have been enacted into law. (Objective 5)

_____ 23. A recent study conducted for the National Council of State Boards of Nursing has demonstrated that most graduates can immediately assume full staff nurse responsibilities. (Objective 7)

_____ 24. The scope of practice for the professional and that for the technical nurse are clearly defined and differentiated. (Objective 7)

_____ 25. Most nursing theories have little applicability to the actual practice of nursing. (Objective 10)

Matching Questions

Match the numbered terms with the lettered statements.

A. 1. National League for Nursing (Objective 3)

2. State Board of Nursing (Objective 3)

   3. National Federation of Licensed Practical Nurses (Objective 3)

   4. American Nurses Association (Objective 2)

   5. North American Nursing Diagnosis Association (Objective 3)

       ____ a. Developed a position paper on nursing education

       ____ b. Has the responsibility for accrediting nursing programs

       ____ c. Is the organization that has developed nursing diagnoses

       ____ d. Is the organization that licenses nurses

       ____ e. Is the organization for licensed practical nurses

Match each numbered theory with its author.

  B. 1. Unitary man

      2. Adaptation

      3. Self-care concept

      4. Interpersonal relationships

      5. Health care systems model (all Objective 9)

       ____ a. Sister Callista Roy

       ____ b. Hildegard Peplau

       ____ c. Martha Rodgers

       ____ d. Betty Newman

       ____ e. Dorothy Orem

Match the title of each study, paper, or proposal with the organization or political body that sponsored it.

  C. 1. *Toward Quality in Nursing*

      2. *A Position Paper on Educational Preparation for Nurse Practitioners and Associates to Nurses*

      3. *Defining and Differentiating ADN and BSN Competencies*

      4. *A Study of Nursing Practice and Role Delineation and Job Analysis of Entry-Level Performance of Registered Nurses*

      5. *Registered Care Technologist* (all Objective 2)

       ____ a. American Nurses Association

       ____ b. National Council of State Boards of Nursing

       ____ c. Surgeon General's Consultant Group in Nursing

       ____ d. American Medical Association

       ____ e. Midwest Alliance in Nursing (MAIN)

Multiple-Choice Questions

_____ 1. A study that was published in the 1950s and had a significant impact on nursing was the
- a. Goldberg report.
- b. Surgeon General's report.
- c. Flexner report.
- d. Brown report.

(Objective 1)

_____ 2. The Brown report recommended that nursing education
- a. move away from the system of apprenticeship that predominated at the time.
- b. be federally funded.
- c. require master's degrees of all faculty.
- d. limit admissions to the nursing classes.

(Objective 1)

_____ 3. The Brown Study was conducted
- a. right after World War I.
- b. right after World War II.
- c. after the Korean conflict.
- d. after the Vietnam conflict.

(Objective 1)

_____ 4. The Surgeon General's report recommended that
- a. more financial assistance be provided for nursing education.
- b. roles of variously prepared graduated be differentiated.
- c. more studies be conducted on the nursing shortage.
- d. associate degree nursing programs be closed.

(Objective 1)

_____ 5. The accreditation standards for the Council of Associate Degree Programs now stipulate that nurse educators possess a
   a. diploma in nursing.
   b. baccalaureate degree in nursing.
   c. master's degree in nursing.
   d. doctorate in nursing.
   (Objective 2)

_____ 6. The Surgeon General's Report emphasized
   a. the need for changes in nursing education.
   b. the need for better prepared faculty.
   c. the changing role of the nurse.
   d. the need for more nurses.
   (Objective 2)

_____ 7. The ANA position paper on nursing education was published in
   a. 1940.
   b. 1965.
   c. 1973.
   d. 1985.
   (Objective 3)

_____ 8. Which of the following was based on the belief that improvement of nursing practice depended on the advancement of nursing education?
   a. The ANA position paper
   b. The Surgeon General's report
   c. The Brown report
   d. The Goldmark report
   (Objective 3)

_____ 9. The ANA position paper was developed by the
   a. Committee on Education.
   b. Committee on Economic Welfare.
   c. Committee on Accreditation.
   d. Committee on Standards of Education.
   (Objective 3)

10. The organization that developed the 1965 position paper on nursing education was the
    a. NLN.
    b. ANA.
    c. Nurses Association of the American College of OB/GYN.
    d. Association of Nurse Anesthetists.
    (Objective 3)

11. Which of the following statements accurately reflects one of the four positions taken in the ANA position paper?
    a. All of the current forms of nursing education should be continued.
    b. All education for nursing should occur in 4-year schools.
    c. The education for all who practice nursing should take place in institutions of higher education.
    d. The education of assistants in health care should be discontinued.
    (Objective 3)

12. The ANA position paper advocated which one of the following degrees or certificates as mandatory for entry into professional practice?
    a. Master's degree
    b. Bachelor's degree
    c. Associate degree
    d. Diploma
    (Objective 3)

13. Which of the following is one of the assumptions on which the ANA position paper is based?
    a. There will be a decrease in the number of nurses needed.
    b. Education for nursing has expanded as far as it can go.
    c. No other health occupation workers are needed to function as assistants to nurses.
    d. The professional practitioner is responsible for the nature and quality of all nursing care that patients receive.
    (Objective 3)

14. The first state to adopt a resolution regarding the entry-into-practice issue was the state of
   a.   New York
   b.   California
   c.   Texas
   d.   Arkansas
   (Objective 3)

15. The ANA position paper presented many concerns. Among them was the concern for
   a.   mobility for nurses.
   b.   job placement.
   c.   articulated nursing programs.
   d.   recruitment of faculty.
   (Objective 4)

16. Which state now requires a baccalaureate degree in nursing in order to write the registered nursing licensing examinations?
   a.   California
   b.   Washington
   c.   North Dakota
   d.   New Hampshire
   (Objective 4)

17. Among the first organizations to support the position of the ANA on nursing education was the
   a.   NLN.
   b.   National Student Nurses Association.
   c.   National Federation of Licensed Practical Nurses.
   d.   American Hospital Association.
   (Objective 3)

_____ 18. One of the major problems associated with the ANA position paper is related to

    a.   the salary of nurses.

    b.   the rights of nurses to bargain collectively.

    c.   the continuing education of nurses.

    d.   the titling of graduates of the different programs.

    (Objective 4)

_____ 19. Which of the following statements is true of the grandfather clause?

    a.   The grandfather clause has been a standard feature that allows persons to continue to practice their profession after new qualifications are enacted into law.

    b.   The grandfather clause was mandated in legislation passed when the Supreme Court reached a decision on the Galt case.

    c.   The grandfather clause is applicable to blue-collar occupations but not to nursing.

    d.   The grandfather clause will expire by the year 1994, so nursing should make any needed changes soon.

    (Objective 5)

_____ 20. A feature that allows persons to continue to practice their profession after new qualifications that they might not meet have been enacted into law is known as a (an)

    a.   waiver.

    b.   grandfather clause.

    c.   immunity clause.

    d.   granted release.

    (Objective 5)

_____ 21. The process by which nurses licensed in one state can gain licensure in another state without reexamination is commonly termed

    a.   transferability.

    b.   protractability.

    c.   extendibility.

    d.   interstate endorsement.

    (Objective 6)

22. Which of the following skills is most likely to be expected of all nurses of tomorrow?
    a.   Ability to perform venipuncture
    b.   Ability to read electrocardiogram strips
    c.   Ability to apply fetal monitors
    d.   Ability to operate a computer
    (Objective 7)

23. One method proposed for recognizing differentiated practice would be through
    a.   additional licensure.
    b.   career ladders.
    c.   continuing education.
    d.   simulated clinical testing.
    (Objective 7)

24. One of the major challenges facing nursing today is the task of
    a.   setting accreditation standards.
    b.   attracting men into the profession.
    c.   describing and differentiating the competencies of graduates of various programs.
    d.   establishing faculty work loads.
    (Objective 7)

25. Nursing in the future may well require that all nurses possess
    a.   the ability to speak at least two languages.
    b.   understanding of accounting principles.
    c.   computer literacy.
    d.   calculus skills.
    (Objective 8)

_____ 26. One of the changes we are beginning to see in nursing education is the advent of programs that have been designed to

    a.   meet the needs of the adult learner.

    b.   provide for greater structure in the program of learning.

    c.   make more electives available to students.

    d.   move students more rapidly through the program.

    (Objective 8)

_____ 27. A significant change in nursing practice is the trend toward

    a.   community-based practice.

    b.   the use of all-registered nurse staffing.

    c.   the revival of the functional nursing approach.

    d.   longer hospital stays.

    (Objective 8)

_____ 28. Nursing educators are revising programs of study to address the needs of

    a.   economically disadvantaged students.

    b.   hospital administration.

    c.   the new high school graduate.

    d.   the adult learner.

    (Objective 8)

_____ 29. One of the major concerns facing nursing education today is that of

    a.   budget constraints.

    b.   lack of public support for nursing.

    c.   oversupply of qualified faculty.

    d.   recruitment of students.

    (Objective 8).

_____ 30. The bill that has made federal dollars available to nursing education is the
    a. Social Security Act.
    b. Taft-Hartley Act.
    c. Nurse Training Act.
    d. Buckley Amendment.
    (Objective 9)

_____ 31. Which one of the following individuals developed a theory of nursing built around the concept of adaptation?
    a. Martha Rodgers
    b. Betty Neuman
    c. Dorothy Orem
    d. Sister Callista Roy
    (Objective 11)

_____ 32. The nursing theory that has been used by the North American Nursing Diagnosis Association is a (an)
    a. adaptation model.
    b. systems model.
    c. interpersonal model.
    d. energy fields model.
    (Objective 11)

_____ 33. Which one of the following individuals developed a theory of nursing around the concept of self-care?
    a. Martha Rodgers
    b. Betty Neuman
    c. Dorothy Orem
    d. Sister Callista Roy
    (Objective 11)

4 | Credentials for Health Care Providers

Purpose

This chapter acquaints students with the various credentials used by individuals in the health care field. The discussion includes credentials in nursing, the history of their development, and the role that credentials play in the profession. It explores nursing licensure, what it means, who controls it, and how it affects the individual who wishes to practice nursing. Issues surrounding the use of additional credentials such as certification are also discussed.

Objectives

1. Define and discuss the concept of credentialing.

2. Differentiate between a diploma, certification, and licensure as credentials.

3. Explain the concepts of permissive and mandatory licensure for practice.

4. Outline the history of nursing licensure.

5. Identify the major content areas in laws regulating nursing practice.

6. Outline the role of the State Board of Nursing.

7. Discuss the process of revocation of a nursing license.

8. Differentiate between licensure by examination and licensure by endorsement.

9. Discuss the historical development of the licensing examination for nursing.

10. Discuss current trends in nursing licensure.

11. Describe the role of the Commission on Graduates of Foreign Nursing Schools.

12. Discuss the concept of certification in nursing.

13. Explain the problems associated with certification in nursing.

Key Terms

Board of Nursing

certification

computerized adaptive
    testing (CAT)

computerized simulation
    testing (CST)

credential

license

licensure

licensure by endorsement

mandatory licensure

NCLEX-PN

NCLEX-RN

Nurse Practice Act

permissive licensure

revocation

Situations to Foster Critical Thinking

1. Several nurses on your unit would like to see a change made in the Nursing Practice Act in your state. You have been asked to gather information regarding the steps that should be taken to initiate a change. Where would you begin? Who would you write or telephone? Give the rationale for why you included the persons or organizations you have identified. How long might you expect the process to take? (Objectives 5, 6)

2. Do you believe the Nurse Practice Act for your state should include provisions for expanded practice? Provide a rationale for your answer. If you believe it should not, what group do you believe should oversee expanded practice? Why? Provide a rationale for your answer. (Objectives 5, 6, 12).

3. Grace Barker is completing the registered nurse program at Rio Santiago College in California. She plans to get married and move with her husband to Illinois. She plans to work until he completes his medical residency. What options are available to Grace with regard to securing a license in Illinois? Which option would you advise her to pursue? What is the rationale for your answer? Where should she write or call for information? (Objectives 6, 8)

4. Now that licensing examinations are computerized, do you think computerized simulation testing (CST) will be adopted in the future? What would you see as the benefits of CST? (Objective 10)

5. As an associate degree graduate, you have been on a medical unit for 15 months. It is your goal to specialize in obstetrics. What steps would you take to begin this process? Would you seek additional formal education? Why or why not? How would you pursue a transfer to the obstetric unit of the hospital? From which professional organization would you seek certification? Provide the rationale for your decision. (Objectives 12, 13)

Discussion/Essay Questions

1. Why are credentials for members of health occupations important to the public? (Objective 1)

2. What credentialing mechanisms are used by some allied health professions? (Objective 1)

3. Explain the difference between a license and a certificate. (Objective 2)

4. What is certification and what are its advantages as a credentialing method? (Objective 2)

5. Anyone who provides health care to the public should be licensed by the state. Agree or disagree with this statement and provide the rationale for your position. (Objectives 2, 3)

6. What are the benefits of mandatory licensure for nursing? (Objective 3)

7. What do you believe to be the most significant event in the history of nursing licensure? Why? (Objective 4)

8. Identify the major topics usually included in the Nurse Practice Act and discuss how these affect nursing practice. (Objective 5)

9. Describe how rules and regulations relate to the state law regulating nursing? (Objective 5)

10. On what grounds might your license as a registered nurse be revoked? (Objective 7)

11. How are graduates of foreign nursing schools admitted to practice in the United States. (Objective 11)

12. Define certification. (Objective 12)

13. What problems are associated with certification in nursing and how might these affect you in the future? (Objective 13)

Fill-In-The-Blank Questions

1. The two purposes of regulating the practice of any health occupation are to _____ and to _____. (Objective 1)

2. Licensure is controlled by the _____ but certification is usually controlled by _____. (Objective 2)

3. The organization that originally began the effort to license nurses was the _____. (Objective 3)

4. _____ licensure is a system whereby an individual may choose to become licensed to provide evidence of competence, but a license is not required to practice. (Objective 3)

5. The first state to pass a mandatory licensure law for registered nurses was _____.(Objectives 3, 4)

6. Some states require completion of _____ to renew a health care license. (Objective 4)

7. The _____ campaigned vigorously for the adoption of state licensure laws. (Objective 4)

8. North Dakota is the first and only state to require a _____ degree for registered nursing. (Objective 4)

9. The organization that originally began the effort to license nurses was the _____. (Objective 4)

10. Three common concepts included in the definition of nursing found in nurse practice acts are _____, _____, and _____ _____. (Objective 5)

11. Laws regulating nursing are carried out through _____ and _____. (Objective 5)

12. Model nurse practice acts have been developed by the _____ and the _____. (Objective 5)

13. The Board of Nursing is responsible for developing _____ and _____, which become part of the law. (Objective 6)

14. Two types of disciplinary action may be taken by boards of nursing are _____ and _____. (Objectives 6, 7)

15. The process of obtaining a second license in another state is called licensure by _____. (Objective 7)

16. The current nursing licensure examination is called the _____. (Objectives 9, 10)

17. A computerized licensure examination that presents different questions to different test takers based on their responses to initial questions is called _____. (Objective 10)

18. The purposes of the CGFNS examination are to _____ and _____. (Objective 11)

19. Two organizations that provide certification in a field of nursing are _____ and _____. (Objective 12)

20. The degree most commonly required for certification as a clinical specialist is the _____. (Objective 13)

True-False Questions

_____ 1. The primary purpose of credentialing health care providers is to protect the public. (Objective 1)

_____ 2. Licensure and certification mean the same thing in nursing. (Objective 2)

_____ 3. The credential that is most actively sought by health care providers is licensure. (Objectives 2, 3)

_____ 4. Mandatory licensure means that one must have a license to practice as a registered nurse. (Objective 3)

_____ 5. The state legislative body is responsible for nursing licensure laws. (Objectives 3, 6)

_____ 6. One of the majors goals of the Nurses Associated Alumnae of the United States and Canada was licensure for nurses. (Objective 4)

_____ 7. The first licensure for nurses was introduced in 1865. (Objective 4)

_____ 8. The movement for nursing licensure was begun by Florence Nightingale. (Objective 4)

_____ 9. The Nurse Practice Act spells out the scope of practice. (Objective 5)

_____ 10. Nurse practice acts in all states identify the same steps in the nursing process and give them the same name. (Objective 5)

_____ 11. Definitions of practical (vocational) nursing are less restrictive than those for registered nursing. (Objective 5)

_____ 12. Current nursing licensure laws are the same in all states in the United States. (Objectives 5, 6)

_____ 13. In some states one Nurse Practice Act covers both practical (vocational) nursing and registered nursing. (Objectives 5, 6)

_____ 14. Nurse practice acts contain provisions that may allow those who are not licensed to act as nurses in specific situations. (Objective 5)

_____ 15. All changes in the law are grandfathered. (Objectives 5, 10)

_____ 16. Conviction of a drug-related crime is a reason for revocation of a nursing license in most states. (Objective 7)

_____ 17. The NCLEX-RN examination is based on research that identifies the essential safe behavior of the beginning nurse. (Objective 8)

_____ 18. Once one has obtained a nursing license in any state, it will never be necessary to take the basic licensing examination again. (Objective 8)

_____ 19. All states require a passing score on a comprehensive examination but do not name the examination in the law. (Objectives 9, 10)

_____ 20. In some states license renewal requires only payment of a fee. (Objective 10)

_____ 21. All applicants seeking licensure as a practical or registered nurse should participate in a formal review course. (Objective 10)

_____ 22. Computerized examinations began in 1992 in all states. (Objective 10)

_____ 23. Graduates of foreign nursing schools must take the CGFNS examination in their own countries before coming to the United States. (Objective 11)

_____ 24. All certification for nurse practitioners requires a master's degree. (Objective 12)

_____ 25. All nursing organizations are united in providing certification through a single credentialing center. (Objective 13)

Matching Questions

Match the numbered terms with the lettered definitions.

A.   1. Permissive licensure (Objective 4)

   2. Mandatory licensure (Objective 4)

   3. Certification (Objective 12)

   4. Credential (Objective 1)

   5. Diploma (Objective 2)

   _____ a. Any official document that attests to one's status or abilities

   _____ b. A system that provides for legal recognition of those in a profession who wish to have it

   _____ c. A system that requires those in a profession to have legal recognition of their qualifications

   _____ d. A method by which a profession identifies ability and attests to a person's qualifications to practice

   _____ e. A written certificate attesting to educational attainment

B.   1. Accreditation

   2. Certificate

   3. Credential

   4. Diploma/degree

   5. License

   _____ a. Written proof of one's qualifications to carry out specific activities

   _____ b. Usually granted on completion of an educational program and the passing of a standardized examination

   _____ c. Usually recognizes completion of a designated program of study such as high school

_____ d.   A legal credential

_____ e.   Status awarded to an organization when specified standards have been met (Objectives 1, 2)

Multiple-Choice Questions

_____ 1.   Which of the following is true regarding the concept of credentialing?

   a.   Credentials are written proof of qualifications.
   b.   Credentials always provide legal verification of competence to
practice.
   c.   There are but a few types of credentials.
   d.   Credentials are awarded only by the State Board of Nursing.
   (Objective 1)

_____ 2.   Which of the following are professionals who are licensed in all
states?

   a.   Physicians, psychologists, pharmacists, and nurses
   b.   Psychologists, pharmacists, dentists, and nurses
   c.   Physicians, dentists, psychologists, and nurses
   d.   Physicians, dentists, pharmacists, and nurses
   (Objectives 1, 2)

_____ 3.   Which of the following statements is true of the credentialing of
health occupations?

   a.   Most health occupations are now credentialed through a national voluntary system.
   b.   There are national criteria that states use to determine whether
or not a given occupation should be licensed.
   c.   Each state has acted independently which (if any) health occupations must be credentialed.
   d.   All health occupations are required to demonstrate competence
through continuing education.
   (Objective 1)

____ 4. One of the arguments against having professional groups accredit programs in their own area of expertise is
   a. loss of objectivity.
   b. cost.
   c. lack of skilled accreditors.
   d. lack of standards.
   (Objectives 1, 2)

____ 5. Licensing differs from credentialing in that licensing
   a. is not revokable.
   b. is more costly.
   c. confers a legal status.
   d. is recognized nationally in all health professions.
   (Objective 2)

____ 6. One of the methods through which specialized preparation is recognized in health care is
   a. certification.
   b. accreditation.
   c. verification.
   d. validation.
   (Objective 2)

____ 7. Who usually grants certification?
   a. State agency
   b. Professional organization
   c. Employing institution
   d. None of the above
   (Objective 2)

____ 8. Who grants a license to practice?
   a. State agency
   b. Professional organization
   c. Employing institution
   d. College or university
   (Objectives 2-4)

____   9.   Which of the following is a requirement of mandatory licensure?

   a.   Meeting the established standards

   b.   Graduating from an accredited program

   c.   Being of legally responsible age

   d.   Listing one's name and credentials with a registry

   (Objective 3)

____   10.   Some who oppose permissive rather than mandatory licensure believe that

   a.   it will be more difficult to keep track of where nurses are employed.

   b.   the state will lose revenue from licensure fees.

   c.   patients may be jeopardized by potentially lower-quality care.

   d.   it could result in a shortage of nurses.

   (Objective 3)

____   11.   A license law that permits nurses either to practice without a license or obtain a license is called

   a.   compulsory.

   b.   comprehensive.

   c.   permissive.

   d.   mandatory.

   (Objective 3)

____   12.   Which factor contributed most to uniformity of standards for registration of nurses throughout the United States?

   a.   The pressure of the public for uniformity

   b.   Federal legislation

   c.   National accreditation of schools

   d.   Demands of hospitals for adequately prepared nurses

   (Objective 4)

_____ 13. Which was the first state to enact mandatory licensure for registered nurses?

    a.   Washington

    b.   Ohio

    c.   New York

    d.   Illinois

    (Objective 4)

_____ 14. The legal guide to the practice of registered nursing is the

    a.   ANA Code of Ethics.

    b.   Nightingale Pledge.

    c.   state practice act.

    d.   Patient's Bill of Rights.

    (Objective 5)

_____ 15. The definitions of nursing included in laws regulating nursing practice

    a.   differentiate between baccalaureate and associate degree practice.

    b.   define the scope of practice.

    c.   support master's preparation for beginning practice.

    d.   mandate continuing education.

    (Objective 5)

_____ 16. Major content areas in laws regulating nursing practice include purpose, definitions, and

    a.   licensure fees.

    b.   role of the medical examining committee.

    c.   listing of approved schools.

    d.   qualifications for licensure.

    (Objective 5)

____ 17. The role of the Board of Nursing includes establishing standards for licensure, enforcing disciplinary codes, regulating specialty practice, and

    a. approving nursing education programs.

    B. determining sites for education programs.

    c. approving master's and doctoral programs in nursing.

    d. establishing working conditions for nurses employed in hospital settings.

    (Objective 6)

____ 18. What is the common responsibility of the State Board of Nursing as established by the licensure laws?

    a. Establish essential content for curricula in nursing schools

    b. License health care institutions

    c. Negotiate nurses' salaries

    d. Write the licensing examination

    (Objective 6)

____ 19. What is a common responsibility of the State Board of Nursing identified in the Nurse Practice Act?

    a. Set standards for nursing care

    b. Discipline individuals who have violated provisions of the Nurse Practice Act

    c. Choose future members of the board

    d. Provide specialty certification

    (Objective 6)

____ 20. Which of the following is true regarding nursing licensure?

    a. It is active throughout a lifetime.

    b. It can be revoked under certain circumstances.

    c. It requires retaking the examination if you move from one state to another.

    d. It requires that all applicants be high school graduates.

    (Objectives 6, 7, 10)

____ 21. If you were licensed in Iowa and wished to accept a nursing position in Chicago, Illinois you would

    a.   practice using the Iowa license.

    b.   apply to the state of Illinois to take the Illinois licensing examination.

    c.   apply to the state of Illinois for interstate endorsement.

    d.   apply to the state of Iowa for transfer of your license to Illinois.

(Objective 8)

____ 22. The common state requirements for licensure as a registered nurse include

    a.   United States citizenship.

    b.   graduation from an NLN-accredited school.

    c.   a baccalaureate degree.

    d.   a passing score on the licensure examination.

(Objectives 8-10)

____ 23. The purpose of the licensing examination is to

    a.   differentiate levels of excellence.

    b.   demonstrate basic safe practice.

    c.   establish information to be used for admission to graduate schodl.screen and limit the number of registered nurses.

(Objective 10)

____ 24. A future trend in nursing licensure may be

    a.   computerized adapted testing.

    b.   computerized simulated testing.

    c.   paper/pencil testing.

    d.   oral examinations.

(Objective 10)

25. Which of the following is true regarding computerized adapted testing?
    a. Candidates know immediately whether they have passed or failed.
    b. It presents the same questions to all candidates.
    c. It presents the same questions in a situation format.
    d. It evaluates each response and then selects an appropriate question to present next.

    (Objective 10)

26. The role of the Commission on Graduates of Foreign Nursing Schools (CGFNS) includes
    a. establishing fees for foreign graduates.
    b. assisting foreign graduates with English comprehension.
    c. preparing foreign graduates to take the NCLEX for registered nursing.
    d. investigating and validating credentials held by graduates of foreign nursing schools.

    (Objective 11)

27. Which of the following statements is true of certification?
    a. Certification is a type credentialing that has professional status.
    b. Certification is a type of credentialing that has legal status.
    c. Certification is available only through the ANA.
    d. Certification must always be endorsed by the same Board of Nursing.

    (Objective 12)

28. What process is generally used to recognize specialty training and education in nursing?
    a. Licensure
    b. Certification
    c. Accreditation
    d. Documentation

    (Objective 12)

_____ 29. All certification represents
    a. postbaccalaureate preparation.
    b. master's degree preparation
    c. completion of program of study.
    d. completion of a home study course.
    (Objective 13)

_____ 30. Which of the following statements is true of certification?
    a. All state nursing practice acts recognize certification as a standard for specialty practice.
    b. All hospitals use specialty certification for purposes of establishing salaries and giving promotions.
    c. Certification is understood by the public to represent excellence in practice.
    d. Certification requires that the applicant meet predetermined standards for specialty practice.
    (Objective 13)

_____ 31. Which of the following was the major recommendation of the Study of Credentialing in Nursing?
    a. Eliminate specialized certification
    b. Establish an independent, free-standing center for nursing credentialing
    c. Turn all credentialing over to the professional associations
    d. Move toward institutional licensure
    (Objective 13)

_____ 32. What was the immediate effect of the recommendation of the Study of Credentialing on the credentialing process in nursing?
    a. Credentialing has been moved to the state boards of nursing.
    b. Credentialing is gradually being consolidated under a free-standing credentialing center.
    c. Credentialing is being coordinated by the professional association of nurses.
    d. Study and discussion are continuing.
    (Objective 13)

5 | Legal Responsibilities for Practice

Purpose

This chapter provides a basic foundation for understanding how the law regulates the practice of nursing. The sources of law and how law is administered are explained to enhance the student's understanding of negligence, malpractice, and liability. Specific situations and legal cases pertinent to liability are presented along with suggestions for preventing legal actions.

Objectives

1. Differentiate between the terms ethics and law.

2. Identify two general sources of law and describe their differences.

3. Explain the role of institutional policies and protocols in legal decision-making.

4. Differentiate between civil law and criminal law.

5. Describe some situations in which nurses may be involved in criminal law.

6. Define negligence, torts, and malpractice.

7. Define liability, identifying situations in which liability is shared by employers or supervisors.

8. State points to be considered in the purchase of professional liability insurance.

9. List the most commonly recurring legal issues in nursing.

10. Explain how informed consent, advance directives, and the Patient Self-Determination Act support the patient's rights.

11. Discuss the nurse's responsibility in the specific issues that can constitute malpractice.

12. Identify factors that contribute to a suit being instituted against a health care professional.

13. Discuss a variety of actions by nurses that might prevent the initiation of a lawsuit.

14. *Explain the various aspects of testifying for a legal proceeding.*

Key Terms

advance directive
claims brought insurance
claims occurred insurance
common law
court
criminal law
deposition
discovery
durable power of attorney
durable power of attorney
    for health care
guardian
informed consent
liability

liability insurance
malpractice
minor
negligence
Patient Self-Determination
    Act
privileged communication
regulatory law
res ipsa loquitur
respondeat superior
statutory law
suit
testimony
tort

Situations to Foster Critical Thinking

1. Explain what is meant by the statement "Your professional responsibilities rest on a dual framework of legal and ethical constraints." How do ethics influence our professional practice? Give an example of an instance in which ethics affect our actions as nurses. Give an example of an instance in which our actions are affected by both ethical and legal considerations. Give an example of a situation having both ethical and legal concerns in which the two are divergent. (Objective 1)

2. You have been working for 6 months in a small community hospital that has very limited visiting hours—2—4 pm and 7—9 pm. You believe that the patients would respond better to a more liberal visitation policy. You do not believe, as do some of the nurses and physicians, that this is disruptive to the care routine. How would you go about seeking a change in this policy? What group within the hospital develops the policy? Who enforces it? What strategies might be used to make the change? (Objective 3)

3. You have just received your license to practice as a registered nurse and are employed on the evening shift in a skilled nursing facility. Occasionally you are the charge nurse for that shift.

Today's mail included an unsolicited letter offering you the opportunity to purchase personal liability insurance through your state nurses association for $67 per year. How will you respond to this offer? What information will you need to make a decision? Where will you obtain that information? Why did you respond as you did? (Objective 8)

4. John Miles, a next door neighbor, recently suffered a cardiovascular accident and is now making a slow but positive recovery. However, his wife has been concerned about advance directives as a result of their recent experiences. She has asked you for information on advance directives. Assuming that she knows almost nothing, what information would you provide? What resources would you suggest she contact? What are your legal constraints, if any, in providing this information? Would it be appropriate for you to witness any legal documents that are signed? (Objective 10)

5. You have been asked by your head nurse to prepare a presentation to be shared with other employees on your unit regarding actions nurses can take to prevent the initiation of lawsuits. What would be the most important points you would want to emphasize in the presentation? What resources or resource persons would you contact in your facility? What organizations might you want to contact for information? Where would you begin? (Objectives 12, 13)

6. You are employed as a staff nurse on a telemetry unit. Three months ago a patient on the unit suffered a cardiac arrest after falling from her bed. The family has brought a lawsuit against the hospital, claiming negligence. Although you did not care for the patient, you have received a subpoena to give testimony in the form of a deposition regarding unit protocol. What information do you need? From whom will you obtain that information? When giving your deposition what should you keep in mind? Where will you likely give the deposition? Who can you expect to find in attendance? (Objective 14)

Discussion/Essay Questions

1. What is the difference between common law and statutory law? (Objective 2)
2. How might a court use institutional policy in making a decision about the liability of a nurse in a lawsuit for malpractice? (Objective 3)
3. Give an example of how civil law affects nurses. (Objective 4)
4. Give an example of how criminal law affects nurses. (Objective 4)
5. How is malpractice different from negligence? (Objective 6)
6. What is meant by the term *reasonably prudent nurse*? (Objective 6)
7. When does a nurse have a legal "duty" toward another individual? (Objective 6)

8. How might a court use the concept of a reasonably prudent nurse in making a decision relative to the liability of a nurse in a lawsuit for malpractice? (Objective 7)

9. What is the difference between a liability insurance policy that provides coverage for claims made during the life of the policy and one that provides coverage for incidents that occurred during the life of the policy? (Objective 8)

10. In which situations might false imprisonment be a concern for nurses? (Objective 9)

11. Describe a situation in which the nurse is responsible for obtaining informed consent. (Objective 10)

12. What is meant by defamation of character, and how might a nurse be involved in a legal action with regard to this issue?

13. What constitutes fraud in the practice of nursing?

14. List three instances in which a nurse might have privileged information. (Objectives 11, 12)

15. What are the potential concerns regarding confidentiality when records are computerized? (Objectives 11, 12)

16. Discuss actions a nurse could take to prevent a lawsuit. (Objective 13)

17. What factors might identify a suit-prone patient? (Objective 13)

18. Why is it prudent to have legal counsel before giving a deposition? (Objective 14)

Fill-In-The-Blank Questions

1. Principles of conduct governing one's relationship with others are known as _____. (Objective 1)

2. _____ includes those roles of conduct or action recognized as binding or enforced by a controlling authority such as local, state, or national government. (Objective 1)

3. Law derived from usual practice, such as that seen in policy manuals, is called _____ law. (Objective 2)

4. Law enacted by a legislative body is _____ law. (Objective 2)

5. Enacted laws and regulatory laws fall in the category of _____ law. (Objective 2)

6. Law derived from common usage, custom, and judicial decisions or court rulings is known as _____ law. (Objective 2)

7. Laws relating to crimes against society as a whole make up the body of _____ law. (Objective 4)

8. Laws relating to problems between individuals or businesses that do not affect society as a whole make up the body of _____ law. (Objective 4)

9. Causing injury by failure to behave as a reasonably prudent person is _____. (Objective 6)

10. Causing injury to a person for whom one is responsible by failing to behave as a reasonably prudent professional is _____ _____ ___. (Objective 6)

11. Any time that shared information is detrimental to the person's reputation, the person sharing the information may be liable for _____. (Objective 7)

12. _____ refers to information shared with certain professionals that does not need to be revealed even in a court of law. (Objective 7)

13. _____ transfers the costs of being sued and of any settlement from the individual to a large group. (Objective 7,8)

14. Insurance that covers incidents that occurred while the policy was in force, regardless of when the claim is brought, is known as _____. (Objective 8)

15. The instance in which the employer can be held responsible for the torts committed by an employee is known as _____. (Objective 9)

16. When a nonprofit hospital cannot be held legally liable for harm done to a patient by its employees, it is said to have _____. (Objective 9)

17. The organization that charitable immunity exempts from liability are _____. (Objective 9)

18. One characteristic of the suit-prone patient is that he or she may often be _____. (Objective 12)

19. One action a nurse might take to prevent the initiation of a suit is to ___ _____. (Objective 13)

20. A written legal testimony is called a (an) _____. (Objective 14)

True-False Questions

____ 1. Statutory law derives from common usage, custom, and judicial decisions or court rulings. (Objective 2)

____ 2. Institutional policy is not relevant to a discussion of legal liability. (Objective 3)

____ 3. A violation of civil law can be punished by a jail term. (Objective 4)

____ 4. *Malpractice* is a term used for a specific type negligence. (Objective 6)

_____ 5. The standard of the reasonably prudent nurse applies to the student nurse. (Objective 6)

_____ 6. Liability means that one is legally responsible for what occurs. (Objective 7)

_____ 7. A supervisor is always responsible when an employee is negligent. (Objective 7)

_____ 8. Nurses do not need to purchase professional liability insurance because no one sues a person who has no insurance. (Objective 8)

_____ 9. It is possible for a nurse who restrains a patient in a bed without a medical order to be charged with false imprisonment. (Objective 9)

_____ 10. It is not legal for a nurse to provide a court with information regarding a conversation with a patient. (Objective 9)

_____ 11. Patients who constantly find fault and criticize care are rarely the individuals who file lawsuits. (Objective 13)

_____ 12. There is nothing one can do to prevent malpractice suits. (Objective 13)

_____ 13. A deposition requires the same standard of truthfulness as required when one is testifying in court. (Objective 14)

Matching Questions

Match the numbered terms with the lettered statements:

1. Fraud
2. False imprisonment
3. Battery
4. Assault
5. Slander
6. Libel (all Objective 9)

_____ a. Oral defamation of character

_____ b. Written defamation of character

_____ c. Refusing to allow a person to leave a hospital

_____ d. Threatening to touch a person in an unwanted manner

_____ e. Touching a person in an unwanted manner

_____ f. Deliberate deception for personal gain

Multiple-Choice Questions

_____ 1. Statutory law consists of two categories. One contains those laws enacted by legislative bodies such as a city council or state legislature. The other includes rules and regulations established by
   a. Congress.
   b. governmental agencies such as licensing boards.
   C. the Supreme Court.
   d. local municipalities.
   (Objective 2)

_____ 2. Which of the following is one of the two general sources of law?
   a. Criminal law
   b. Community law
   C. Statutory law
   d. Constitutional law
   (Objective 2)

_____ 3. Our common law is derived from
   a. laws enacted by legislative bodies.
   b. laws established by governmental agencies.
   c. laws that regulate conduct between private individuals.
   d. usage, custom, and judicial decisions.
   (Objective 2)

_____ 4. What is the major purpose of institutional policies?
   a. To serve as guidelines to protect the institution and its employees from legal difficulties
   b. To form the basis for performance evaluation of employees
   c. To meet Joint Commission on Accreditation of Healthcare Organization standards
   d. To establish in writing the hospital's organization hierarchy
   (Objective 3)

___ 5. Civil law consists of
   a. laws that affect the public welfare as a whole.
   b. laws that regulate conduct between private individuals or businesses.
   c. laws generated from common usage and custom.
   d. laws enacted by legislative bodies.
   (Objective 4)

___ 6. Negligence consists of
   a. doing what one should not have done.
   b. not taking action that one should have taken.
   c. breaking the laws relevant to professional practice.
   d. causing injury by failing to act as a reasonably prudent person.
   (Objective 6)

___ 7. Failure to act as a reasonably prudent person would have acted in a specific situation is known as
   a. intentional tort.
   b. malpractice.
   c. negligence.
   d. liability.
   (Objective 6)

___ 8. The nursing student is expected to perform to which standard?
   a. Reasonably prudent person
   b. Reasonably prudent nursing student
   c. Reasonably prudent nurse
   d. There is no standard for nursing students.
   (Objective 6)

___ 9. Being legally responsible for the outcome of an action is referred to as
   a. liability.
   b. responsibility.
   c. intentional tort.
   d. negligence.
   (Objective 7)

____ 10. If you assign tasks to a nursing assistant, are you usually legally liable for whether those tasks were done correctly?

    a. Never

    b. Occasionally, but not usually

    c. Yes

    d. Situations vary so much that you would need legal advice on each individual situation.

    (Objective 7)

____ 11. Could assets held by you and your spouse jointly be claimed by an individual receiving a judgment against you in a malpractice suit?

    a. Not under any circumstances

    b. Yes, in certain states

    c. Only if you are head of a household

    d. Only if you own at least 51% of the assets

    (Objective 8)

____ 12. Fraud is defined as

    a. attempting to hide covert actions.

    b. misunderstanding the truth.

    c. charting incorrectly.

    d. deceiving deliberately for the purpose of personal gain.

    (Objective 9)

____ 13. The patient's having given informed consent means that the patient

    a. totally accepted the plan of the treatment.

    b. clearly understood the choices being offered.

    c. had an opportunity to discuss alternatives with the family.

    d. got a second opinion before signing papers.

    (Objective 9)

14. If a nurse in an emergency situation were to give a patient the lifesaving medicine she believed the physician would order if the physician were present to order it, the nurse would be
    a. acting under the Good Samaritan Act.
    b. guilty of violating the Medical Practice Act.
    c. guilty of violating the Narcotics Act.
    d. assuming expected independence and critical decision-making roles.
    (Objective 9)

15. Which of the following contributes most to suits being filed?
    a. Any error no matter how small
    b. Failure to perceive psychological needs
    c. Serious illness
    d. Incomplete documentation
    (Objective 12)

16. One of the most significant things you can do, as a nurse, to prevent malpractice claims against you is to
    a. carry malpractice insurance.
    b. avoid caring for suit-prone patients.
    c. check with a supervisor before initiating any action.
    d. work at improving your own nursing practice.
    (Objective 13)

17. If you are called to testify in court in your capacity as a registered nurse, it is wise to remember that
    a. you should answer only the questions asked.
    b. you need not tell the entire truth.
    c. you are protected by the Good Samaritan statutes.
    d. you will always be considered an expert witness.
    (Objective 14)

6 | Ethical Concerncs in Nursing Practice

Purpose

This chapter provides a basis for understanding ethical decision-making and the concepts pertinent to that process. It also discusses factors affecting decision-making and how ethics relate to the practice of nursing.

Objectives

1. *Explain how personal religious and philosophical viewpoints, the Code for Nurses, and the Patient's Rights document are used as bases for ethical decision-making.*

2. *Analyze the relationships between basic ethical concepts in ethical decision-making.*

3. *Describe four ethical theories that may be used when considering ethical problems.*

4. *Explain how sociocultural factors affect ethical decision-making for nursing.*

5. *Discuss the various occupational factors that influence decision-making.*

6. *Outline a framework for ethical decision-making.*

7. *Discuss how ethics relate to commitment to the patient/client, commitment to personal excellence, and commitment to nursing as a profession.*

8. *Review the ethical and legal obligations related to the chemically impaired nursing colleague.*

Key Terms

authoritarian	duty
autonomy	ethics
beneficence	fidelity
chemical dependency	justice
deontology	natural law

nonmaleficence

paternalistic

social equity

teleology

utilitarianism

values clarification

veracity

Situations to Foster Critical Thinking

1. The Code for Nurses was written in 1973. Review the document. Do you believe it is current for today's practice? Provide the rationale for your response. If you were going to add or delete content, what would it be? Again provide a rationale for your response. (Objective 1)

2. Compare and contrast the four ethical theories presented in the text. Select the one theory that best accommodates your values. Provide a rationale for selecting that theory as a basis for ethical decision-making. Does that theory have any particular weakness? (Objective 3)

3. Denise Martin is employed as charge nurse in a local nursing home. Recently a decision was made to discontinue the tube feedings a comatose patient has been receiving. Some of the staff, particularly the nursing assistants, are very distressed about this order. What can Denise do to assist her staff? Who might help with the problem? How should she begin? What factors will she need to consider? (Objectives 1, 4, 7)

4. In health care we sometimes do harm to individuals although that is not intended (nonmaleficence). Identify some clinical situations in which this can occur? What will you do as a professional nurse the limit the occurrence of these situations? How will you deal with those that cannot be prevented? (Objective 6)

5. Select a particular ethical issue. Identify how you will address that issue and maintain your personal commitment to excellence. (Objective 7)

6. You have been working on the unit for six months. Recently you have noticed that a colleague has demonstrated difficulty meeting schedules and deadlines, has done sloppy charting, has had two medications errors of which you are aware, and has had four absences in the last month. Several of the patients also have complained that the pain medication they received did not help their discomfort. What would you think might be the problem? What would you do? Where would you begin? Explain why you chose to take the actions you have outlined? (Objective 8)

Discussion/Essay Questions

1. Give examples (anonymous) of situations of which you are aware that pose ethical dilemmas in health care. (Objective 1)

2. What is the purpose of the American Nurses Association Code for Nurses? (Objective 1)

3. Describe a situation in which beneficence and autonomy might be in conflict. (Objective 2)

4. Define the concept of justice from an ethical standpoint. (Objective 2)

5. Do you believe that beneficence, autonomy, or justice has the strongest claim? Why? (Objective 2)

6. Explain how the decision of an individual using utilitarian ethics would differ from that of an individual taking a position that there are consistent moral truths. (Objective 3)

7. Give an example of how using Rawls' approach to social justice might affect an ethical decision. (Objective 3)

8. How does the law affect ethical decision-making? (Objective 4)

9. How have science and technology influenced ethical problems in health care? (Objective 4)

10. How has the paternalistic background of the hospital affected nurses as decision-makers in ethical situations? (Objective 5)

11. Outline a method of self-evaluation that you would feel comfortable using. (Objective 6)

12. Do you believe that nurses should evaluate peers or that evaluation should be performed by supervisors only? Why? (Objectives 7)

13. How might you respond to a negative personal evaluation of your nursing performance? (Objective 7)

14. What should you do if you believe a colleague in nursing is coming to work under the influence of alcohol? (Objective 8)

15. What resources are available in your community and state to assist a chemically dependent nurse? (Objective 8)

Fill-In-The-Blank Questions

1. _____ is a process that includes assessing, exploring and determining personal values. (Objective 1)

2. The _____ of the individual have been increasingly emphasized in all aspects of living and, more recently, in dying. (Objective 1)

3. The obligation to do good, not harm, to other people is known as ____ _____. (Objective 2)

4. The right to make one's decision is termed _____. (Objective 2)

5. The obligation to be fair to all people is termed _____. (Objective 2)

6. _____ refers to the obligation to be faithful to the agreements and responsibilities that one has undertaken. (Objective 2)

7. A moral principle or a set of moral principles that can be used in assessing what is morally right or morally wrong is a (an) _____ . (Objective 2)

8. The ethical theory that states that an act is right if it is useful in bringing about a desirable or good outcome for the greatest number is _____ __. (Objective 3)

9. Rawl's approach to justice focuses on the concept of _____ __ _____. (Objective 3)

10. Relationships among nurses who work together in which they support one another, share in decision making, and present a unified approach to problems are called _____ relationships. (Objective 5)

11. Two factors in the background of hospital governance have contributed to nurses not being decision makers. These two factors are _____ and _____. (Objective 5)

12. Making a severely critical remark to a patient about a physician 's practice could result in a legal charge of _____. (Objective 7)

13. Stealing a small amount or stealing objects of little value is known as _____. (Objective 7)

14. The first step in any situation in which you believe substandard care exists is to _____. (Objective 7)

True-False Questions

____ 1. Deciding to participate in providing care for clients who are having abortions is primarily an ethical issue rather than a legal issue. (Objective 1)

____ 2. Values clarification is a process of assessing, exploring, and determining one's own personal values. (Objective 1)

____ 3. The ANA Code for Nurses is legally binding. (Objective 1)

____ 4. The International Council of Nurses Code for Nurses is not used by nurses in the United States because there is a national code in the United States. (Objective 1)

____ 5. The rights outlined in the American Hospital Association's A Patient's Bill Of Rights identifies penalties for hospitals that fail to ensure patients these rights. (Objective 1)

_____ 6. The American Hospital Association's Patient'sBill of Rights is legally binding on all hospitals that are members of that association. (Objective 1)

_____ 7. Beneficence refers to the obligation to do good and not harm. (Objective 2)

_____ 8. Justice means that all people should be treated equally. (Objective 2)

_____ 9. Autonomy refers only to the rights of the patient to self-determination. (Objective 2)

_____ 10. The size of the group being affected by ethical decision has little to do with the decision-making process. (Objective 4)

_____ 11. The value a society places on the individual or the family directly influences the standard of care. (Objective 4)

_____ 12. A culture's religious values and belief in an afterlife directly affect ethical issues. (Objective 4)

_____ 13. The judicial system has little impact on ethical decision-making. (Objective 4)

_____ 14. Collective bargaining contracts can protect nurses in making ethical decisions. (Objective 5)

_____ 15. Today, nurses are seldom represented on hospital ethics committees. (Objective 5)

_____ 16. The paternalistic background of the hospital has supported nurses as decision makers. (Objective 5)

_____ 17. The authoritarian background of the hospital has limited nurses as decision makers. (Objective 5)

_____ 18. Nurses demonstrate commitment to excellence by participating in ethics committees. (Objective 7)

_____ 19. Nurses are seldom in the position of being asked to recommend a physician or other type of care provider. (Objective 7)

_____ 20. A final alternative to a problem in your work setting is to offer your resignation if the change is not made. (Objective 7)

Matching Questions

Match the numbered terms with the lettered statements.

A. 1. Justice

2. Veracity

3. Beneficence

    4. Autonomy

    5. Fidelity

        ____ a. The obligation to do good not harm to people

        ____ b. The right to make one's own decisions

        ____ c. The obligation to be fair to all people

        ____ d. The obligation to be faithful to the agreements and responsibilities that one has undertaken

        ____ e. Telling the truth (all Objective 2)

B. 1. Social equity and justice

    2. Utilitarianism

    3. Natural law

    4. Deontology

        ____ a. An act is right if it is useful in bringing about a good outcome or end.

        ____ b. An ethical theory based on a concept of moral duty or obligation

        ____ c. Actions are morally right when they are in accord with our nature and end as human beings.

        ____ d. An approach to ethics that supports the person most disadvantaged by the situation
(all Objective 3)

Multiple-Choice Questions

____ 1. Which of the following statements is true of ethical concerns in nursing?

    a. Nurses are not expected to make ethical decisions.

    b. Correct ethical decisions are outlined in the ANA Code for Nurses.

    c. Increasing technology has resulted in situations for which there are no clear-cut answers.

    d. Nurses are participants in all ethical decisions that affect their practice.

(Objective 1)

_____ 2. What a patient can expect in care is often found in documents identifying the patient's rights. Guidelines for specific ethical professional practice are often found in

    a.   accreditation standards.

    b.   utilization reviews.

    c.   position papers.

    d.   codes of ethics.

    (Objective 1)

_____ 3. One method used to help assess, explore, and determine our personal values is through the process of

    a.   meditation.

    b.   mediation.

    c.   consciousness raising.

    d.   values clarification.

    (Objective 1)

_____ 4. A common guideline accepted by the profession as a whole for nurses to use in making ethical decisions is

    a.   the Hippocratic Oath.

    b.   the Morse code.

    c.   the ANA Code for Nurses.

    d.   the _Encyclopedia of Bioethics._

    (Objective 1)

_____ 5. The Patient's Bill of Rights was written by the

    a.   American Medical Association.

    b.   American Hospital Association.

    c.   American Nurses Association.

    d.   Department of Health and Human Services.

    (Objective 1)

____ 6. The Code for Nurses was developed by
   a. The National League for Nursing.
   b. The National Student Nurses Association.
   c. The American Medical Association.
   d. The American Nurses Association.
   (Objective 1)

____ 7. The obligation to be faithful to the agreements and responsibilities one has undertaken is known as the concept of
   a. veracity.
   b. fidelity.
   c. beneficence.
   d. justice.
   (Objective 2)

____ 8. A nurse believes that the primary consideration in working with a group of patients is that any decision must be fair to all. This attitude represents support of the concept of
   a. beneficence.
   b. autonomy.
   c. justice.
   d. utility.
   (Objective 2)

____ 9. A nurse believes that it is very important to let the patient make his or her own decisions. This attitude represents support of the concept of
   a. beneficence.
   b. autonomy.
   c. justice.
   d. utility.
   (Objective 2)

_____ 10. A nurse believes that the most important consideration is that no harm be done to the patient. This attitude represents support of the concept of

    a. beneficence.

    b. autonomy.

    c. justice.

    d. utility.

    (Objective 2)

_____ 11. The ethical theory that supports the concept that an act is right if it is useful in bringing about a good outcome is the theory of

    a. utilitarianism.

    b. deontology.

    c. natural law.

    d. social equity and justice.

    (Objective 3)

_____ 12. What is the original position according to Rawls?

    a. Being in charge of one's own destiny

    b. Understanding the consequences of one's decisions

    c. Viewing the situation without knowing which one of the participants is yourself

    d. Seeing the situation from the perspective of knowing the outcome

    (Objective 3)

_____ 13. A decision to use available funds to help the greatest number, regardless of seriousness of illness or need, would be most consistent with which philosophical position?

    a. Utilitarianism

    b. Categorical imperative of Kant

    c. Social justice

    d. None of the above

    (Objective 3)

14. One group of individuals that is demanding greater involvement in all aspects of health care is made up of
    a. consumers.
    b. third-party payers.
    c. hospital medical staffs.
    d. nurse practitioners.
    (Objective 4)

15. Which of the following cultural attitudes or situations have affected ethical decision-making?
    a. Emphasis on the community as a consumer unit in health
    b. Media that communicate specific situations to large groups
    c. Values placed on individual autonomy
    d. All of the above
    (Objective 4)

16. What is the major effect that increasing scientific knowledge and technology in health care have had on ethical decision-making?
    a. Decisions may now be made by computers, which are impartial.
    b. Greater technology allows us to put off decisions about death because it can be forestalled.
    c. More complex procedures have all been accompanied by complex ethical concerns.
    d. No basic changes in the ethical questions in health care have been caused by technology.
    (Objective 4)

17. Historically nurses, most of whom are women, have been relegated to dependent and subservient roles due to:
    a. collective bargaining contracts.
    b. their unwillingness to be involved.
    c. the lack of men in nursing.
    d. the authoritarian and paternalistic attitudes of physicians and hospitals.
    (Objective 5)

18. Which of the following most affects the ability of nurses to be autonomous decision makers regarding ethical questions?
    a. Status of the employee
    b. Lack of specific courses in ethics in the basic program
    c. Limited involvement in situations that require ethical decisions
    d. The collegial support of other nurses
    (Objectives 5, 7)

19. Which of the following factors impinges on the nurse's autonomy in ethical decision-making?
    a. Authoritarian background of hospitals
    b. Consumer involvement in health care
    c. Status as an employee
    d. All of the above
    (Objectives 5, 7)

20. In identifying the ethical problem, you will first determine:
    a. what decision must be made.
    b. who will make the decision.
    c. when you must make the decision.
    d. why you need to make a decision.
    (Objective 6)

21. Which of the following responses to a request for recommendation would be ethically and legally appropriate?
    a. Dr. James is a honey—and cute, too.
    b. Dr. Madison is a terror. I wouldn't let him take care of my dog, much less my child.
    c. Dr. Johnson does not usually encourage parent participation in care while a child is hospitalized.
    d. No doctor is as good as Dr. Wilson.
    (Objective 7)

_____ 22. The appropriate way to report poor medical care is first to
   a. confront the physician personally.
   b. discuss your concerns with your immediate supervisor.
   c. tell the client you believe she or he has been the recipient of poor care.
   d. notify the chief of the medical staff in writing.
   (Objective 7)

_____ 23. When you observe an error in nursing care by a peer, an appropriate first action is to
   a. submit a written report to your immediate supervisor.
   b. speak with the nurse privately about your concern.
   c. correct the mistake, but say nothing.
   d. ignore the situation; each nurse is responsible for her or his own practice.
   (Objective 7)

_____ 24. What is the first step in self-evaluation?
   a. Gathering data
   b. Identifying problems
   c. Asking for feedback from others
   d. Setting up a plan for continuing education
   (Objective 7)

_____ 25. A method of evaluating nursing care by examination of records only is called
   a. quality assurance.
   b. audit.
   c. peer review.
   d. accreditation.
   (Objective 7)

26. Criteria that describe the result of care as seen in the patient are
    a. process criteria.
    b. detail criteria.
    c. evaluation criteria.
    d. outcome criteria.
    (Objective 7)

27. Criteria that describe the correct actions to be taken by health care providers are
    a. process criteria.
    b. detail criteria.
    c. evaluation criteria.
    d. outcome criteria.
    (Objective 7)

28. When you suspect that a nursing peer is practicing under the influence of alcohol, you should first
    a. confront the individual personally.
    b. talk with your immediate supervisor in an informal way.
    c. ask to transfer to another unit to avoid legal liability.
    d. record specific dates and behaviors observed.
    (Objective 8)

29. You are working days and have noted that whenever a certain nurse works nights, the postoperative patients complain of unrelieved pain and very restless nights. An appropriate first action would be to
    a. tell the nurse involved what you have observed and that you will be watching the situation closely.
    b. suggest to the head nurse that the nurse in question be transferred to the day shift where more nurses are around to observe her behavior.
    c. document specific dates, patients, drugs given, and patient responses.
    d. tell the head nurse that nurse X is using drugs and should be dismissed.
    (Objective 8)

_____ 30. In addition to concerns that the chemically impaired nurse may injure patients, we are concerned
  a. about the liability of working with someone who is chemically impaired.
  b. on a personal level for the nurse who is afflicted.
  c. about staffing during the time the nurse is left off the unit.
  d. that the Board of Nursing not learn of the problem.
  (Objective 8)

7 | Bioethical Issues in Health Care

Purpose

This chapter exposes the student to some of the many bioethical issues emerging in health care today. Included are topics such as family planning practices, abortion, genetic screening, and surrogate motherhood. The chapter also covers issues related to dying, such as active euthanasia and passive euthanasia, the problems related to securing organs for donations, and informed consent and treatment. The chapter concludes with a discussion of the treatment of the mentally ill.

Objectives

1. *Define bioethics and give reasons nurses need to have some understanding of bioethical concerns.*

2. *Discuss the history of family planning practices in the United States and identify positions people take related to family planning practices, including abortion.*

3. *Discuss the arguments some people have against the Human Genome Project and its relationship to genetic screening.*

4. *List some of the possible ethical and legal problems associated with the practice of employing a surrogate mother.*

5. *Discuss the problems associated with determining when death has occurred.*

6. *Review and examine right-to-die issues, differentiating between active euthanasia and passive euthanasia.*

7. *Discuss the major issues related to withholding or withdrawing treatment and patients' rights with regard to informed consent and treatment.*

8. *Identify major concerns associated with organ transplantation.*

9. *Discuss reasons we have difficulty establishing firm rules regarding treatment of the mentally ill.*

10. *Outline concerns related to the rationing of care.*

Key Terms

abortion	genetics
advance directives	genetic screening
artificial insemination	gene therapy
assisted death	informed consent
behavior control	in vitro fertilization
bioethics	living will
death	organ procurement
durable power of attorney for health care	patient self-determination (PSD)
eugenics	property rights
euthanasia	right to die
negative euthanasia	surrogate mother
positive euthanasia	withdrawing treatment
family planning	withholding treatment
futile treatment	

Situations to Foster Critical Thinking

1.   Think of a situation in which you have been involved as a nursing student in which bioethics was a consideration. What information was needed to deal with the situation? Where could that information have been obtained? What was your personal position regarding the issue? How did you reach that position? Was it supported by others? (Objective 1)

2.   You are working the night shift on the obstetrics unit. As you make rounds at 1:30 am, you find Mrs. Rodder, a Roman Catholic patient who has just delivered her 7th child, crying. As you talk with her, you learn that she does not want to go home the next morning because she is afraid she will be pregnant again within the next year. Giving full consideration to her religious views, what will be your response to her concern? (Objective 2)

3.   What social and legal concerns can you identify with regard to the Human Genome Project? What might be the worst situation that could evolve? What might be the best? How might these concerns be mitigated? (Objective 3)

4.   If you were given the assignment of developing guidelines for the practice of using a surrogate mother, what criteria would you establish?

How would you ensure that these criteria were carried out? To whom would you assign this responsibility? (Objective 4)

5. Mr. Allen is preparing for discharge following recovery from a serious heart attack. He and his wife are interested in learning more about durable power of attorney in the event that the family has serious problems in the future. What information would you provide to them? To whom would you refer the family? What would be the major considerations? (Objectives 6, 7)

6. Do you believe the federal government should invest large amounts of money in research related to the development of artificial organs, such as kidneys, hearts, or livers? Give the reasons for your response. If it is yes, how would you propose that this be funded? (Objective 8)

Discussion/Essay Questions

1. Discuss what is meant by the word *bioethics*. (Objective 1)

2. Which bioethical issues cause us the most concern and why? (Objective 1)

3. Why have bioethical concerns increased in the last ten years? (Objective 1)

4. Discuss the position of the Roman Catholic Church on birth control? (Objective 2)

5. How does the age of consent affect decision-making with regard to bioethical issues? (Objective 2)

6. Cite at least two reasons why a family may not wish to practice birth control? (Objective 2)

7. Discuss the arguments in favor of the availability of abortion. (Objective 2)

8. Discuss the arguments against the availability of abortion. (Objective 2)

9. Are there any extenuating circumstances that one who is basically against abortion might consider? If so, what are they?

10. What is artificial insemination and what are the different ways in which it can be carried out? (Objective 2)

11. What is the major reason for performing an amniocentesis? Do you think there are other reasons that are equally important? (Objective 3)

12. What are the advantages and disadvantages of being able to do an amniocentesis? (Objective 3)

13. Identify some of the conditions that can be diagnosed prenatally via amniocentesis. (Objective 3)

14. Define the term *eugenics* and explain when it was first discussed. (Objective 2)

15. Explain how events that occurred during Hitler's regime resulted in eugenics becoming very unpopular. (Objective 3)

16. Give some arguments supporting the use of in vitro fertilization and some arguments against the use of it. (Objective 3)

17. Cite two concerns that arise when a surrogate mother has been employed to give birth to a baby. (Objective 4)

18. Describe death as defined in *Black's Law Dictionary*. (Objective 5)

19. Why is the *Black's Law Dictionary* definition of death no longer adequate to meet the demands of society? (Objective 5)

20. What is currently accepted as a definition of death? (Objective 5)

21. Identify some situations in which persons might support negative euthanasia. (Objective 6)

22. Differentiate between positive euthanasia and negative euthanasia. (Objective 6)

23. What is the purpose of the living will? (Objective 7)

24. What are the rights of the patient with regard to informed consent? (Objective 7)

25. Identify at least one situation in which it would be appropriate to withhold treatment. (Objective 7)

26. How does the concept of withholding treatment differ from that of withdrawing treatment? (Objective 7)

27. Provide a definition of behavior control as it is used in the treatment of the mentally ill. (Objective 9)

28. Why is anything that smacks of behavior control regarded with suspicion in our society? (Objective 9)

29. What are some of the major guidelines that have been proposed for dealing with the area of behavior control? (Objective 9)

30. What is electroconvulsive therapy and why are some persons opposed to it? (Objective 9)

31. How is society dealing with the problem of scarce medical resources? (Objective 10)

32. Outline the concerns related to rationing of care. (Objective 10)

33. If you were responsible for determining who would receive care and to what degree, what criteria would you use for making your decisions? (Objective 10)

Fill-In-The-Blank Questions

1. _____ is the study of ethical issues that result from technological and scientific advances. (Objective 1)

2. In 1893, Congress passed the Comstock Act prohibiting the sale, mailing, or importation of any drug or article that _____. (Objective 2)

3. A clear legal concept of planned parenthood was not developed until _____ when the Supreme Court established the right of the individual to obtain medical advice about contraception.

4. The age at which one is capable of giving deliberate and voluntary agreement is known as the _____.

5. A youth who is sufficiently mature and intelligent to understand the nature and consequences of a treatment that is for her or his benefit is termed a (an) _____. (Objective 2)

6. When a pregnancy is deliberately interrupted for medical reasons, the abortion is referred to as (an) _____. (Objective 2)

7. The court case that resulted in the legalization of abortion is known as the _____ decision. (Objective 2)

8. A technique in which approximately 20 mL of fluid is withdrawn from the amniotic sac in the uterus of a pregnant woman is called _____ _____. (Objectives 2, 3)

9. The movement devoted to improving the human species through the control of hereditary factors in mating is known as _____. (Objective 3)

10. The practice by which a woman agrees to bear a child conceived through artificial insemination and to relinquish the baby at birth to others for rearing is known as _____. (Objective 4)

11. When the husband's sperm is used for artificial insemination of his wife, it is known as _____ insemination. (Objective 4)

12. Until recently, the most widely accepted definition of death was from _____. (Objective 5)

13. Literally translated, the term *euthanasia* means _____. (Objective 6)

14. Withholding treatment could be considered _____ euthanasia. (Objective 7)

True-False Questions

____ 1. *Bioethics* is sometimes also called *biomedical ethics*. (Objective 1)

____ 2. Bioethical issues surrounding the delivery of health care are always clear and straightforward. (Objective 1)

____ 3. The Catholic Church believes strongly that the natural use of reproductive powers ensures the propagation of the race. (Objective 2)

_____ 4. The age at which one may consent to treatment and the age at which one can refuse treatment are the same. (Objective 2)

_____ 5. The legal aspects of abortion were not clarified until January 1983. (Objective 2)

_____ 6. There will be times when physicians' ethical and moral convictions prevent them from complying with certain aspects of care. (Objective 2)

_____ 7. Abortion is the termination of pregnancy before viability of the fetus. (Objective 2)

_____ 8. No one objects to abortion when it terminates a pregnancy that results from rape or incest. (Objective 2)

_____ 9. With increasing frequency, voluntary sterilizations have been requested by couples for purposes of terminating reproductive ability. (Objective 2)

_____ 10. Artificial insemination is a newly introduced procedure. (Objective 2)

_____ 11. One major disadvantage of amniocentesis is that it cannot be done until the 36th week of gestation. (Objective 3)

_____ 12. One obvious outcome of amniocentesis is that a woman carrying a defective fetus has the option of seeking an abortion. (Objective 3)

_____ 13. Eugenics is the movement devoted to improving the human species through genetic control. (Objective 3)

_____ 14. Newer definitions of death have been built around the concept of human potential. (Objective 5)

_____ 15. There have been no statements or positions issued with regard to withdrawing or withholding treatment. (Objective 7)

_____ 16. The steps to be taken when an individual remains in a persistent vegetative state are clear and straightforward. (Objective 7)

_____ 17. Physicians are in agreement about how much patients should know about their condition. (Objective 7)

_____ 18. In many ways, the ability to use organs for transplantation has required a clearer definition of death. (Objective 8)

_____ 19. The patient is the only one who can give permission for the removal of organs at the time of death. (Objective 8)

_____ 20. In many states citizens are being asked to make informed decisions about the rationing of health care. (Objective 10)

Matching Questions

Match the numbered terms with the lettered statements.

A. 1. Emancipation of a minor (Objective 2)

2. Informed consent (Objective 7)

3. Paternalism (Objective 7)

4. Age of consent (Objective 2)

5. Mature minor (Objective 2)

_____ a. The age at which one is capable of giving deliberate and voluntary agreement

_____ b. A youth who is sufficiently mature and intelligent to understand the nature and consequences of a treatment

_____ c. Entire surrender by the parents of the right to care for, have custody of, and take earnings of a child

_____ d. The right to know what treatment will be administered

_____ e. The locus of decision-making is moved from the patient to the physician.

B. 1. Negative euthanasia (Objective 6)

2. Positive euthanasia (Objective 6)

3. Negative eugenics (Objective 3)

4. Positive eugenics (Objective 3)

_____ a. The elimination of unwanted characteristics from a population by discouraging "unworthy" parents

_____ b. The increase of desirable traits in a population by urging "worthy" parents to have children

_____ c. A situation in which medication is administered to hasten death

_____ d. A situation in which no heroic measures are taken to prevent death

Multiple-Choice Questions

_____ 1. The study of ethical issues that result from technological and scientific advances is known as

a. biometrics.

b. bioethics.

c. biophysics.

d. biogenesis.

(Objective 1)

_____ 2.   Biomedical ethics
    a.   is a subdiscipline of a larger area of the philosophical study of morality.
    b.   provides definitive answers about what is right and what is wrong in medical practice.
    c.   is a discipline that has a long history.
    d.   is fairly narrow in scope.
    (Objective 1)

_____ 3.   The first writings expressing concern about our growing population were written in
    a.   1560.
    b.   1600.
    c.   1798.
    d.   1850.
    (Objective 2)

_____ 4.   Among the religions that forbid the use of artificial birth control is that of the
    a.   Jews.
    b.   Free Methodists.
    c.   Southern Baptists.
    d.   Roman Catholics.
    (Objective 2)

_____ 5.   Central to all discussions of contraception is the issue of
    a.   the greatest good for the greatest number.
    b.   the overpopulation of the world.
    c.   the freedom to control one's body.
    d.   the rights of the unborn infant.
    (Objective 2)

_____   6.   The major factor influencing how an individual may choose to practice contraception is that person's

   a.   age.

   b.   sex.

   c.   values.

   d.   heritage.

   (Objective 2)

_____   7.   At one time it was believed that children could tell right from wrong and had reached the age of reason by the age of

   a.   5.

   b.   7.

   c.   10.

   d.   15

   (Objective 2)

_____   8.   Under the concept of a mature minor, a minor who wants access to birth control devices

   a.   must first secure his or her parents' permission.

   b.   must demonstrate ability to pay for them.

   c.   must promise not to share them with friends.

   d.   may obtain them on request.

   (Objective 2)

_____   9.   Regarding the care of minors, the most liberal legislation applies to

   a.   the treatment of venereal disease.

   b.   the prescribing of birth control.

   c.   the birth of children.

   d.   the setting of broken bones.

   (Objective 2)

_____ 10. In 1973 a Model Act, which addresses the issue of consent of minors for health care, was developed by
   a.   the Fellows of the College of OB/GYN.
   b.   the Academy of Family Practitioners.
   c.   the American Academy of Pediatrics.
   d.   the American Psychiatric Association.
   (Objective 2)

_____ 11. Conservatives argue against sex education and the dispensing of contraceptives by the schools on the basis that it
   a.   is unsafe.
   b.   is immoral.
   c.   is too costly.
   d.   erodes the role of the family.
   (Objective 2)

_____ 12. The age of consent refers to
   a.   the age at which one may vote.
   b.   the age at which one may purchase alcoholic beverages.
   c.   the age at which one may witness legal documents.
   d.   the age at which one is capable of giving deliberate and voluntary agreement.
   (Objective 2)

_____ 13. If an abortion is done to save the life of the mother, that abortion is termed
   a.   spontaneous
   b.   therapeutic.
   c.   complete.
   d.   elective.
   (Objective 2)

_____ 14. Central to people's concerns about the ethics of abortion are their beliefs about
   a. life after death.
   b. passive euthanasia.
   c. when life begins.
   d. the value of life.
   (Objective 2)

_____ 15. Abortions were first legalized in the United States in 1973 following a decision by
   a. the United States Supreme Court.
   b. the New York State Supreme Court.
   c. the Vatican.
   d. the Institute of Society, Ethics, and Life Sciences.
   (Objective 2)

_____ 16. The concept based on the principle that it is wrong to give birth to a child whose life will not have the same quality as that of other children is known as
   a. negative eugenics.
   b. wrongful birth.
   c. wrongful death.
   d. positive eugenics.
   (Objective 2)

_____ 17. One of the arguments against programs of genetic screening is that they
   a. are considered normal.
   b. can lead to a downfall of a nation.
   c. can place a great deal of strain on a marriage.
   d. exceed the bounds of what human beings should "tamper with."
   (Objective 3)

___ 18. The science of improving the physical and mental qualities of human beings by controlling factors that influence heredity is known as
   a. euthanasia.
   b. bioethics.
   c. cloning.
   d. eugenics.
   (Objective 3)

___ 19. Negative eugenics advocates
   a. elimination of unwanted characteristics from a nation by discouraging "unworthy" parents from having children.
   b. increasing desirable traits in the population by urging "worthy" parents to have children.
   c. taking no extraordinary measures to sustain life.
   d. taking steps to hasten the individual's death.
   (Objective 3)

___ 20. The project that has as one of its goals the detailed mapping of genetic make-up is known as the
   a. Behavioral Response project.
   b. Project Fifteen.
   c. Genetic Determination Project.
   d. Human Genome Project.
   (Objective 3)

___ 21. A goal of genetic research would be to
   a. identify defective fetuses so that they could be aborted if the family wished.
   b. identify and isolate defective genes and replace them with functional genes.
   c. describe genetic make-up.
   d. provide a rationale for the practice of eugenics.
   (Objective 3)

_____ 22. The practice by which a woman agrees to bear a child conceived through artificial insemination and to relinquish the baby at birth to others for rearing is known as

    a. in vitro fertilization.

    b. surrogate motherhood.

    c. adoption.

    d. family planning.

    (Objective 4)

_____ 23. Until recently, the most widely accepted definition of death was from

    a. the Old Testament.

    b. the United States Constitution.

    c. the Hippocratic Oath.

    d. *Black's Law Dictionary.*

    (Objective 5)

_____ 24. Newer definitions of death have been built around the concept of human potential. The method most often used to assess this capability is

    a. the computed tomography scan.

    b. the electroencephalogram.

    c. the electrocardiogram.

    d. magnetic resonance imaging.

    (Objective 5)

_____ 25. The definition of brain death is also used in the process of

    a. seeking power of attorney.

    b. notifying next of kin.

    c. obtaining organs for transplantation.

    d. removing valuables.

    (Objective 5)

_____ 26. Which one of the following statements is true of our definition of death?
   a.   All parts of the body die simultaneously.
   b.   The moment of death is unmistakable.
   c.   The absence of brain waves over a given period of time is a generally accepted definition of death.
   d.   Only after respirations have ceased for a period of 8 hours can the body be considered legally dead.
   (Objective 5)

_____ 27. A patient who has given informed consent
   a.   has totally accepted the plan of the treatment.
   b.   clearly understands the choices being offered.
   c.   participated in planning the treatment to be administered.
   d.   solicited a second opinion before signing papers.
   (Objective 7)

_____ 28. One of the major bioethical issues facing Americans today is
   a.   where to invest research dollars.
   b.   the feasibility of germ warfare.
   c.   the acquisition and allocation of scarce medical resources.
   d.   the rising cost of medical insurance.
   (Objectives 8, 10)

_____ 29. One of the problems highlighted by the need for donated organs is

   a.   the cost of organ removal.
   b.   identification of the sex of the person donating the organ.
   c.   who is responsible for approaching the family.
   d.   whether the organ should be transported out of state.
   (Objective 8)

30. When giving consideration to ethical concerns regarding behavior control, a major consideration is
    a. identifying what constitutes deviant behavior.
    b. the age of consent.
    c. the religious preference to the client.
    d. the type of condition from which the client suffers.
    (Objective 9)

8 | The Health Care Delivery System

Purpose

This chapter presents the basic structure of the health care delivery system. The roles of the various health care providers are discussed. Concerns related to the distribution of resources and power in the system are explored.

Objectives

1. *Explain the role of the primary health care provider and identify the individuals who fulfill this role.*

2. *Describe the roles of the various allied health care workers.*

3. *Describe the differences between institutions that provide acute care and those that provide long-term care.*

4. *Compare the various community health care agencies that provide care.*

5. *Discuss the ways in which alternative health care resources meet health care needs.*

6. *Describe the different mechanisms of health care financing.*

7. *Explain how regulatory agencies, payers, providers, and consumers demonstrate power in the health care system.*

8. *Describe economic influences on health care delivery.*

Key Terms

alternative health care
  resource
community mental health
  centers
diagnosis-related group
  (DRG)
health maintenance
  organization

insurance company
long-term care facility
Medicaid
Medicare
managed care
nurse practitioner
nursing home

occupational therapist

occupational therapy
    assistant

physical therapist

preferred provider
    organization (PPO)

primary care provider

respiratory therapist

Situations to Foster Critical Thinking

1. Most of the proposals for a reformed health care system involve greater use of a primary care physician as a "gatekeeper" to specialist care. What are the benefits to the system of this approach? What are the problems associated with this approach? Weighing the benefits and problems, take and support a position for or against the use of the primary physician as a "gatekeeper".

2. Outline the advantages and disadvantages of licensing all individuals who perform the various diagnostic procedures. How would it change relationships in the health care system if a license were not required to perform these procedures?

3. A multidisciplinary team for a home care agency may be led by the nurse, the physical therapist, or the social worker. Develop a set of criteria that could be used by the agency to determine which professional should be the team leader for an individual client.

4. An acute care hospital is opening a subacute care unit designed to care for individuals who are expected to need care for 15 to 90 days after their acute hospital stay. These individuals are expected to be discharged home. If you are asked to work on this unit, what questions should you ask about staffing patterns, care delivery approach, accountability and responsibility, and relationships with the rest of the facility? What questions should you ask regarding your own status as an employee?

Discussion/Essay Questions

1. List at least three different occupations that could be considered primary health care providers and explain why you included them. (Objective 1)

2. Discuss the differences between the physician's assistant and the nurse practitioner. (Objective 1)

3. Why are some physicians opposed to nurse practitioners? (Objective 1)

4. Identify a health occupation in which there are both technologists and technicians and explain the education and responsibilities of each. (Objective 2)

5. Identify a health occupation in which there are both therapists and therapy technicians and explain the education and responsibilities of each. (Objective 2)

6. Identify a health maintenance organization in your community. (Objective 4)

7. What is a preferred provider organization (PPO)? Identify a PPO in your community. (Objective 6)

8. How does a home health care agency differ from a public health department? (Objective 4)

9. Where are shortages of primary care providers most apparent and why? (Objective 1)

10. What are the reasons a person might consult a folk medicine healer rather than a conventional health care provider? (Objective 5)

11. What group has traditionally had the most power in the health care system? Do you see any changes in this occurring in your community? If so, describe them. (Objective 7)

12. Why is cost containment a major concern in health care? (Objective 8)

13. How does cost containment affect the delivery of nursing care? (Objective 8)

14. What are DRGs and how are they related to the prospective payment system? (Objective 6)

Fill-In-The-Blank Questions

1. A health care professional who provides initial entry into the health care delivery system is called a _____. (Objective 1)

2. Some people have suggested that nurse practitioners not be independently licensed but instead be considered _____. (Objective 1)

3. The highest-level title among those working in allied health fields is usually _____. (Objective 2)

4. The agency that is usually responsible for monitoring and maintaining the health of the general population is the _____. (Objective 4)

5. There is a shortage of physicians in _____ areas of the United States. (Objective 1)

6. One reason why people seek out alternative health care providers is the _____ nature of the interactions these individuals maintain. (Objective 5)

7. The health care discipline that has traditionally had the most power in the system is _____. (Objective 7)

8. Cost containment measures have resulted in more care being delivered _____ the hospital. (Objective 8)

9. The categories used to determine payment under Medicare are called _____. (Objective 6)

True-False Questions

____ 1. Only a physician can be a primary health care provider. (Objective 1)

____ 2. Nurse practitioners are unable to charge high enough fees to pay for malpractice insurance if it costs them as much as it costs physicians. (Objective 8)

____ 3. The terms *technician* and *technologist* have a legally established meaning. (Objective 2)

____ 4. Community mental health agencies are able to meet the needs of all persons with mental illness who do not need hospitalization. (Objective 4)

____ 5. Alternative health care resources have clearly been shown to provide no objective improvement in any person's health status. (Objective 5)

____ 6. The most powerful group in the health care system has traditionally been the physicians. (Objective 7)

____ 7. Cost containment has resulted in a shortage of hospital beds. (Objective 8)

____ 8. Diagnosis-related groups are simply a classification system used to determine payment for health care services. (Objective 6)

Multiple-Choice Questions

____ 1. The person who furnishes entry into the health care system is generally known as a

a. primary health care provider.

b. primary nurse.

c. family practitioner.

d. referring physician.

(Objective 1)

____ 2. Primary health care providers are best described as

    a. persons who furnish entry into the health care system.

    b. persons assigned to a group of patients in the hospital.

    c. physicians called for a consultation.

    d. insurance companies, such as Blue Cross, that help pay medical bills.

(Objective 1)

____ 3. The term *primary health care provider* refers to

    a. the type of nursing care given in hospitals.

    b. the first physician a patient ever sees.

    c. a person who furnishes entry into the health care system.

    d. a health care organization that provides care at a low cost.

(Objective 1)

____ 4. One of the problems related to nurses working in expanded roles is

    a. whether such nurses should be classified as physician's assistants.

    b. the problems of third-party payment.

    c. credentials required for practice.

    d. all of the above.

(Objective 1)

____ 5. Which of the following statements is true of the physician's assistant (PA)?

    a. All PAs must have completed a baccalaureate program.

    b. All PAs must be licensed in the state in which they practice.

    c. All PAs must work under the direction of a physician.

    d. All of the above.

(Objective 1)

____ 6. Which of the following phrases best describes a technologist?

    a. An individual with good on-the-job training

    b. An individual with baccalaureate preparation

    c. An individual with an associate degree in an allied health field

    d. An individual with postbaccalaureate preparation

(Objective 2)

_____ 7. One of the phenomena exhibited in the health care delivery system in the last 10 to 20 years has been

a. an increase in the incidence of communicable disease.

b. a decrease in the incidence of chronic illness.

c. an increase in the number of different health occupations.

d. a decrease in demand for preventive health services.

(Objective 2)

_____ 8. To assist in containing the cost of health care, the federal government has subsidized the creation of

a. osteopathic hospitals.

b. nontraditional approaches to health care.

c. health maintenance organizations.

d. emergency care centers.

(Objective 6)

_____ 9. The agency that is primarily concerned with setting hospital standards is the

a. National League for Nursing.

b. Department of Health and Human Services.

c. state rate commission.

d. Joint Commission on Accreditation of Healthcare Organizations.

(Objective 7)

_____ 10. Which of the following statements is true of long-term care facilities?

a. They must all have accreditation.

b. They include nursing homes and centers for developmentally disabled adults.

c. They care for persons with acute episodes of chronic illness.

d. They all receive funding from the federal government under Title VI.

(Objective 3)

____ 11. The health care institution charged with the responsibility of maintaining the health of the community as a whole is the

    a. community mental health center.

    b. public health department.

    c. visiting nurse agency.

    d. health maintenance organization.

    (Objective 4)

____ 12. What is one of the major benefits that health maintenance organizations offer over other health care providers?

    a. They are more personal.

    b. They tend to emphasize preventive care.

    c. They are all well located for availability to all.

    d. The client can always have a choice of care providers.

    (Objective 6)

____ 13. Nursing homes and convalescent centers are

    a. acute care facilities.

    b. community health care facilities.

    c. alternative health care facilities.

    d. long-term care facilities.

    (Objective 3)

____ 14. Where is there still an inadequate supply of primary health care providers?

    a. Suburban areas

    b. Urban areas

    c. Rural areas

    d. All of the above

    (Objective 1)

_____ 15. What is one major factor that may prompt people to seek an alternative health care system?

    a. Lack of money

    b. The belief system of the individual

    c. Unavailable of conventional care alternatives

    d. Pressure from the media

    (Objective 5)

_____ 16. Which of the following circumstances would be most likely to result in a person seeking an alternative health care system?

    a. No one in the conventional agencies is able to provide a cure.

    b. A patient believes that no one in the conventional agency cared about him or her as an individual.

    c. The person was informed about potential side effects of medications and treatments.

    d. The family was asked to participate in providing care.

    (Objective 5).

_____ 17. Which group has traditionally had the most power in the health care system?

    a. Physicians

    b. Hospital administrators

    c. Insurance companies

    d. Governmental agencies

    (Objective 7)

_____ 18. What factor contributes most heavily to increasing power for nurses in the health care system?

    a. Nurses are seen in positive light by patients.

    b. Nurses have college educations.

    c. Nurses are the largest single group of health care providers.

    d. Nurses are getting involved in political processes.

    (Objective 7)

19. Which segment of our society has shown the greatest cost increases in the last 15 years?
    a. Food
    b. Housing
    c. Transportation
    d. Health care
    (Objective 8)

20. The most important cause of increases in the cost of health care has been
    a. the effect of raises in nurses' salaries.
    b. the fact that the average patient's stay in the hospital is shorter.

    c. the cost of new technology.
    d. the increased cost of maintenance energies such as heat and lights.
    (Objective 8)

21. Which of the following has contributed to increases in health care costs?
    a. Increases in wages of health care workers
    b. Increases in physicians' charges
    c. The cost of new technology
    d. All of these
    (Objective 8)

22. DRGs set a limit on
    a. the amount of health care a person can receive.
    b. the number of days of hospitalization allowed.
    c. the reimbursement that the hospital will receive for care.
    d. the number of diagnostic tests that may be performed.
    (Objective 6)

_____ 23. What is a prospective payment system?

    a.   One in which the hospital receives payment before the service is provided

    b.   One in which the patient pays in advance for services needed

    c.   One in which the hospital is paid a monthly sum by an insurance company for providing services at a special rate

    d.   One in which the reimbursement amount for care is set ahead of time

(Objective 6)

9 | Collective Bargaining

Purpose

This chapter explores the basic activities related to collective bargaining. Starting with a history of collective bargaining, it focuses on collective bargaining as it is applied in nursing. The language used in collective bargaining is introduced as the various concepts are discussed. The chapter considers the issues that arise when collective bargaining is applied to the nursing profession, especially the controversy that exists with regard to nurses exercising the right to strike. The chapter includes a discussion of the purpose of a grievance process in the contract.

Objectives

1. *Define and use appropriately the terms most commonly associated with collective bargaining.*

2. *Discuss the history of collective bargaining as it applies to nursing.*

3. *Explain the concept of arbitration.*

4. *Identify at least four items that should be included in a contract for nurses.*

5. *Explain the grievance process.*

6. *Discuss the concerns nurses have regarding membership in a collective bargaining group.*

7. *Outline the advantages and disadvantages of having the state nurses' association serve as the bargaining agent for nurses.*

8. *Identify some of the ways shared governance may affect collective bargaining.*

Key Terms

agency shop
authoritative mandate
binding arbitration

collective action division
collective bargaining
common interest bargaining

concession bargaining

contract

deadlock

final offer

grievance process

injunction

lockout

mediation

National Labor Relations Act (NLRA)

National Labor Relations Board (NLRB)

negotiation

professional collectivism

ratify

reinstatement privilege

shared governance

unfair labor practice

union busting

unions

Situations to Foster Critical Thinking

1. The Supreme Court ruled that a group of licensed practical nurses in a nursing home were supervisors according to the definitions of the NLRA because they directed the work of nursing assistants. Therefore, these LPNs were not protected under the NLRA, and had no right to collective bargaining; their dismissal for complaints regarding quality of care was upheld. What are the implications of this ruling for registered nurses in hospitals?

2. Consider that you are working in an acute care hospital that is covered by a collective bargaining contract and the administration decides to restructure the organization. Is this proposal related to rights under the contract? What information do you need to gather to determine this? Which individuals should be involved in decision-making regarding the proposed restructuring?

3. Mary Watkins, RN, works in a hospital that has a policy of placing nurses on probation if they have three medication errors. She notes that many nurses do not fill out quality assurance (QA) reports when medication errors occur; however, she has always been very careful to follow the policy and complete QA reports. She makes a third error and is notified that she is being placed on probation. Would this be grievable under a contract? What questions would she need to ask to determine this? What considerations do you think have a bearing on this case? What would you do if you were in this situation?

4. Jim Nathan, RN, works in a long-term care facility. The nursing assistants are considering establishing a union to bargain with the corporation that owns the facility. Would Jim be part of their union? What should be his role in the process? Provide a rationale for the actions you think he should take?

Discussion/Essay Questions

1. Discuss what is meant by the term *negotiate*. (Objective 1)
2. Why was it once seen as incongruous with values of nursing for nurses to negotiate salaries? Why has that changed? (Objective 2)
3. Briefly outline the history of collective bargaining. (Objective 2)
4. In general, what is the role of the NLRB? (Objective 2)
5. Why were nurses among the last of the professions to be included in national labor laws? (Objective 2)
6. What exceptions to the national laws were made when nurses were included in the laws? Why was it thought that these were necessary? (Objective 2)
7. Define the terms *union, mediate,* and *arbitrate*. (Objective 3)
8. Define the term *collective action division*. (Objective 3)
9. Discuss several activities that could be considered unfair labor practices. (Objective 3)
10. What is the purpose of negotiating an agency shop? (Objective 3)
11. Discuss the role of the mediator and the arbitrator in a collective bargaining situation. (Objective 4)
12. Discuss at least two types of arbitration, explaining how they differ. (Objective 4)
13. What is a contract and why is it desirable to have one? (Objective 5)
14. List at least three items that should be included in a nurses' contract. (Objective 6)
15. Explain the purpose of a grievance process. (Objective 5)
16. How does a grievance differ from a complaint? (Objective 5)
17. Why does the role of the supervisor present problems to nurses from a collective bargaining view point? (Objective 6)
18. Discuss the issues of professionalism versus unionism in nursing. Do you believe it is an issue that is no longer important? (Objective 2)
19. Why are nurses sometimes reluctant to join a bargaining group? (Objective 2)
20. Give some reasons why many nurses believe they are best represented at the bargaining table by the state nurses' association. (Objective 7)
21. Are there reasons why nurses might be better represented at the bargaining table by another group? What problems might this create? (Objective 7)
22. What concerns do most nurses have when a strike is called? (Objective 6)

23. What are some arguments supporting strike activities by nurses? (Objective 6)

24. What provisions should be made to continue care of the community if a strike is called? Do you think there should be these provisions? (Objective 6)

25. What changes did we see in the collective bargaining process in the 1980s? (Objective 2)

26. What is meant by pay equity? (Objective 4)

Fill-In-The-Blank Questions

1. Bargaining or conferring with another party or parties to reach an agreement is called _____. (Objective 1)

2. In the year _____, amendments to the NLRA made it possible for employees of nonprofit health care institutions to bargain collectively. (Objective 2)

3. What party will represent a group at the bargaining table is determined by _____. (Objective 2)

4. An early reformer who generated interest in collective bargaining was _____. (Objective 2)

5. The NLRA passed in 1935 was also known as the _____. (Objective 2)

6. In 1947, the original labor act was amended through the _____, which was also known as the _____. (Objective 2)

7. A set of procedures by which an employee representative and an employer representative negotiate to obtain a signed contract is called _____. (Objective 1)

8. Bargaining or conferring with another party to reach an agreement is referred to as _____. (Objective 1)

9. When a branch of a professional association assumes the responsibility of negotiating contracts for its members, the negotiating group may be known as a (an) _____. (Objective 1)

10. A (An)_____ is any action that interferes with the rights of employees or employers as described in the amended NLRA. (Objective 1)

11. The advantage to a union of having a contract with an agency shop clause is that it _____. (Objective 4)

12. In _____, both parties are obligated to abide by the decision of the arbitrator. (Objective 3)

13. When the parties doing the negotiating cannot come to an agreement on an issue, they are said to be _____ or the two groups are _____ ____ on the issue. (Objective 3)

14. A major criticism of the arbitration process is _____. (Objective 3)

15. Three items that should be included in a contract for nurses are _____ ____, _____, and _____. (Objective 4)

16. The grievance process spells out in _____ a series of steps to be taken to _____ the area of dissension. (Objective 5)

17. A (An) _____ is an allegation by any party functioning under a collective bargaining agreement that a violation of the contract has occurred. (Objective 1)

18. The organizations that have carried out the majority of the collective bargaining activities for nurses are the _____. (Objective 7)

19. A (An) _____ is a guarantee offered to striking employees that they will be rehired after the strike. (Objective 1)

20. When the negotiation process does not go smoothly, the last alternative available to the employee is to _____. (Objective 6)

21. _____ results in an explicit exchange of labor cost for improvement in job security. (Objective 1)

22. Organized nurses in some states have focused their bargaining energies on issues of _____. (Objective 7)

True-False Questions

____ 1. As early as 1850, reformers were interested in collective bargaining issues. (Objective 2)

____ 2. The first national labor policy of the United States was the Wagner Act. (Objective 2)

____ 3. The Wagner Act made it possible for nurses to bargain collectively for salaries. (Objective 2)

____ 4. The role of the NLRB was to ensure that the conditions of labor legislation were properly enforced. (Objective 2)

____ 5. The NLRB has no authority over the elections of union representatives. (Objective 2)

____ 6. The NLRA has never been amended. (Objective 2)

____ 7. Collective action divisions operate under different constraints than do unions. (Objective 2)

____ 8. The NLRB administers the NLRA. (Objectives 2, 3)

_____ 9. The issue of agency shop is one rather frequently agreed on in the negotiation process. (Objective 4)

_____ 10. If a contract is _ratified_, it has been accepted by the members of the bargaining group. (Objective 1)

_____ 11. A mediator may never serve as an arbitrator. (Objective 3)

_____ 12. The final offer approach is a type of binding arbitration. (Objective 3)

_____ 13. A lockout is said to occur when an employer closes a factory or other place of business to make employees agree to terms. (Objective 1)

_____ 14. Reinstatement privileges cannot be offered unconditionally. (Objective 1)

_____ 15. A mediator is a third person who may join the bargainers to assist in the reconciliation of differences. (Objective 1)

_____ 16. Binding arbitration means that both parties are obligated to abide by the decision of the arbitrator. (Objective 3)

_____ 17. Contracts can be enforceable whether written or oral. (Objective 1)

_____ 18. There are no specific criteria for the content to be included in a contract. (Objective 4)

_____ 19. An important part of a contract is the section that establishes the grievance process. (Objective 5)

_____ 20. In the collective bargaining process, supervisors function just as any other member of the employees' group. (Objective 2)

_____ 21. Only nurses may represent nurses at the bargaining table. (Objective 2)

_____ 22. There is only one kind of strike. (Objective 1)

_____ 23. Federal law makes it illegal for nurses to strike. (Objective 2)

_____ 24. The right to bargain collectively was initially a controversial issue among nurses and other members of the health care team. (Objective 2)

Matching Questions

Match the numbered terms with the lettered statements.

A. 1. Collective action division

2. Unfair labor practice

3. Agency shop

4. Lockout

5. Final offer (all Objective 1)

     ____ a. Arbitrator selects the most reasonable package offered

     ____ b. Requires those who do not want to be union members to pay the union fee rather than union dues

     ____ c. Formed when a professional group assumes the responsibility for doing the collective bargaining

     ____ d. Any action that interferes with rights of employees or employers in the bargaining process

     ____ e. Occurs when the employer closes the plant to cause the employees to settle the contract

B. 1. Mediator

   2. Union

   3. Binding arbitration

   4. Authoritative mandates

   5. Collective action division (all Objective 1)

     ____ a. An organized group of employees

     ____ b. A professional organization that does the bargaining for its members

     ____ c. Peaceful settlements encouraged by a high-ranking official

     ____ d. Third person who joins bargainers to reconcile differences

     ____ e. Both parties are obligated to abide by the arbitrator's decision

Match the following numbered statements with the dates.

C. 1. No-strike policy officially adopted by the ANA

   2. First labor policy passed in the United States

   3. Taft-Hartley Act amends the NLRA

   4. Nurses are included in national policies

   5. ANA appointed a committee to study employment conditions (all Objective 2)

     ____ a. 1935

     ____ b. 1945

     ____ c. 1947

     ____ d. 1950

     ____ e. 1974

Multiple-Choice Questions

_____ 1. The term *negotiate* implies
   a. compromise on both parts.
   b. that management has the "upper hand."
   c. that labor can eventually "make a point."
   d. that mediation will be needed to settle the contract.
   (Objective 1)

_____ 2. The Taft-Hartley Act was amended to allow nurses to bargain collectively for salaries and working conditions in
   a. 1935.
   b. 1945.
   c. 1947.
   d. 1982.
   (Objective 2)

_____ 3. The Taft-Hartley Act is also known as
   a. the Wagner Act.
   b. the Labor Management Act.
   c. the NLRA.
   d. Public Law 93-360.
   (Objective 2)

_____ 4. One of the reason why nurses were not included in collective bargaining laws was concern for
   a. the image of nursing.
   b. the effect on physicians.
   c. the effect on health care.
   d. the cost.
   (Objective 2)

_____ 5. The role of the board of inquiry is
    a. fact finding.
    b. mediating.
    c. arbitrating.
    d. conciliating.
    (Objective 1)

_____ 6. Engaging in unfair labor practices may
    a. bring an immediate end to the strike.
    b. jeopardize the individual's right to job reinstatement.
    c. be divided into seven classifications.
    d. result in work stoppages.
    (Objective 2)

_____ 7. A person chosen by agreement of both parties to decide a dispute between them is known as a (an)
    a. mediator.
    b. board of inquiry.
    c. arbitrator.
    d. conciliator.
    (Objective 1)

_____ 8. When a branch of a professional association does the negotiating for its members, the group may be known as
    a. a union.
    b. a closed shop.
    c. an agency shop.
    d. a collective action division.
    (Objective 7)

_____ 9. An agency shop is considered desirable by the employees' group because
    a. it encourages membership in the organization.
    b. it means higher salaries.
    c. it eliminates the cost of arbitration.
    d. it guarantees acceptance of the contract.
    (Objective 4)

____ 10. Binding arbitration implies that both sides
   a. are obligated to abide by the decision of the arbitrator.
   b. may make one final best offer.
   c. can bring new negotiators to the table.
   d. have 10 days to settle their differences.
   (Objective 3)

____ 11. A contract is stronger if it is
   a. written.
   b. negotiated each year.
   c. reviewed by an arbitrator.
   d. recorded in the county courthouse.
   (Objective 1)

____ 12. A good contract includes, in addition to other items, which of the following?
   a. A copy of the bylaws governing the organization
   b. A section establishing guidelines for disciplinary problems
   c. The names of the chief officers of each party
   d. A copy of Public Law 93-360
   (Objective 1)

____ 13. The purpose of a grievance process in a contract is to
   a. differentiate grievances from complaints.
   b. protect the "little guy."
   c. establish a method for adjustment of grievances.
   d. protect the management from "wrongful suits."
   (Objective 5)

____ 14. Grievances must be differentiated from
   a. issues.
   b. complaints.
   c. errors in judgment.
   d. unprofessional behavior.
   (Objective 5)

_____ 15. One of the first concerns faced by nurses as they prepare to bargain collectively is
   a. gaining public support.
   b. passing legislation to make bargaining legal.
   c. supporting the professional image.
   d. selecting a bargaining group to represent them.
   (Objective 7)

_____ 16. One of the advantages of having nurses negotiate for nurses is that
   a. they are a stronger union.
   b. they have been doing negotiations for years.
   c. they have more funds to devote to the activities.
   d. they thoroughly understand the concerns of nurses.
   (Objective 7)

_____ 17. An advantage of having the state nurses' association responsible for the bargaining for nurses is that
   a. this association has more political clout.
   b. it is cheaper.
   c. it is easier to negotiate issues such as those related to patient care.
   d. nurses are more experienced in bargaining.
   (Objective 7)

_____ 18. One argument for having another organization do the negotiating for nurses is that
   a. it is less expensive.
   b. another organization may understand the nuances of bargaining better than nurses.
   c. it will avoid strikes.
   d. it will create a better public image.
   (Objective 7)

_____ 19. The major reason nurses have difficulty conducting a strike is
    a. they don't know how to organize.
    b. they are concerned about interruption of patient care.
    c. the are concerned about being called "scabs" by their colleagues.
    d. they are concerned about recovering their jobs after the strike.
(Objective 2)

_____ 20. The organization that represents the majority of nurses at the bargaining table is
    a. the state nurses' association.
    b. the National League for Nursing.
    c. the Teamsters.
    d. the Federation of Nurses and Heath Care Professionals.
(Objective 7)

_____ 21. Today may nurses are concerned about
    a. pay equity.
    b. the fact that it is illegal to strike.
    c. whether it is professional to strike.
    d. laws preventing collective bargaining by nurses.
(Objective 12)

_____ 22. Concession bargaining is
    a. a process by which there is an explicit exchange of labor costs for improvements in job security.
    b. a process by which each party gives in on critical issues.
    c. a process by which management offers compromises to the union in exchange for longer hours.
    d. a process by which the union requests additional pay for longer hours.
(Objective 12)

10 | The Political Process and Health Care

Purpose

This chapter provides the basis for understanding the political process in general and how it applies to health care. The role of the individual in the political process is emphasized, and specific information is presented on how the individual can participate and influence outcomes. The major federal legislation that has affected nursing in the past and current legislative concerns are presented. Common state and local political concerns are outlined.

Objectives

1. Explain the relevance of the political process to nursing.
2. Discuss seven ways you might influence the political process.
3. Outline the current U.S. federal governmental role to health care.
4. Discuss the various proposals related to a national health care system.
5. Explain common state legislative concerns.
6. Discuss common local political concerns.
7. Identify how politics is relevant to your participation in organizations.

Key Terms

appropriation
authorization
benefit package
budget
health care reform
lobbying
managed competition
Medicaid

Medicare
Occupational Safety and Health Act (OSHA)
peer review
single-payer system
quality assurance
uncompensated care
universal coverage

Situations to Foster Critical Thinking

1. Identify a health care plan. Analyze it in relationship to cost, comprehensiveness, choices, and accessibility.

2. Identify a current health-related issue in your community. Present your own position with regard to this issue with the rationale for your position. Determine where decisions will be made in regard to this issue. Outline the mechanisms you could use to influence decision-making in regard to this issue.

3. Suppose that the Nurse Practice Act in your state will be subject to sunset review at the end of next year. What features of the current law are most important to you? What features would you like to change? What mechanisms are available to you to have input into this process?

4. The Public Health Department of your community is asking for public support for its outreach program for childhood immunization. What actions might you take to support this effort?

Discussion/Essay Questions

1. Identify one issue in which the political process is particularly relevant and explain why you think so. (Objective 1)

2. Define what is meant by the political process and explain how this might apply to an organization. (Objective 1)

3. What is lobbying and how might you participate in lobbying at the state level? (Objective 2)

4. What do you believe would have more effect on a federal legislator—a dozen signed form letters or one personally written letter? Explain your reasoning. (Objective 2)

5. How does the American Nurses Association try to affect political outcomes? (Objective 2)

6. Do you believe the Nurse Education Act should be funded by the federal government? Explain your position. (Objective 3)

7. Discuss the impact of two major provisions of the Nurse Education Act in the past. (Objective 3)

8. Who is covered by Medicare and how is Medicare financed? (Objective 3)

9. Discuss a recent change in the Medicare Act that has affected nursing practice. (Objective 3)

10. What governmental body administers the Medicare funds for families? On what is this based? How does this affect the delivery of nursing care services? (Objective 3)

11. Discuss the purpose of the OSHA and its impact on health care. (Objective 7)

12. What effect could the decreased federal funds for health care planning have on health care within a community? Explain your answer. (Objective 3)

13. One of the provisions of the Maternal Child Health Act was funding for research. How might this have an impact on nursing? (Objective 3)

14. What does catastrophic health coverage usually cover, and how might a decision of the government to provide only this coverage for everyone affect the type of services that nurses would be providing? (Objective 4)

15. When was the Nurse Practice Act in your state last changed? What effect might this have on the activities of your state nurses' association? (Objective 5)

16. What is the major health responsibility of your local government? How might you affect the level of funding for this responsibility? (Objective 6)

17. What is a current major health problem in your community and how are nurses involved in solving it? (Objective 6)

Fill-In-The-Blank Questions

1. Three ways nurses can affect the political process are _____,__ _____, and _____. (Objective 2)

2. The Nurse Education Act provided funding for schools of nursing for _____ and _____. (Objective 3)

3. The two major sections of the Social Security Act that provide care for those over 65 and for dependent individuals are _____ and ____ _____. (Objective 3)

4. The major purpose of OSHA is to _____. (Objective 3)

5. The major purpose of the Maternal-Child Health Act is to _____ _____. (Objective 3)

6. Funds available from the federal government for any health care program must be approved in both an _____ and an _____ act. (Objective 3)

7. To influence the amount of money appropriated for the Nurse Education Act, you should contact your representative when the _____ Act is being considered. (Objective 2)

8. The organization you would join to be a part of the ANA's political action efforts is _____. (Objective 2)

True-False Questions

_____ 1. The political process is a method of influencing decision-making and the allocation of resources. (Objective 1)

_____ 2. The federal government has input into health care only for those receiving Medicare and Medicaid funds. (Objective 3)

_____ 3. The political process consists only of what is done to influence the action of governmental bodies. (Objective 1)

_____ 4. Lobbying is any communication with a government official. (Objective 2)

_____ 5. Nursing organizations have separate but related entities that lobby on issues relevant to nursing. (Objective 2)

_____ 6. When you telephone a legislator, it is preferable to insist that you speak with that individual in person to ensure that your message is communicated. (Objective 2)

_____ 7. The original Nurse Training Act was passed in 1980. (Objective 3)

_____ 8. The Nurse Education (Training) Act has consistently been supported by the presidents of the United States throughout its existence. (Objective 3)

_____ 9. Because there is a shortage of nurses, the Nurse Education Act has been greatly expanded since 1990. (Objective 3)

_____ 10. Medicare serves only those who are 65 years of age and older. (Objective 3)

_____ 11. Support for renal dialysis is included in Medicare. (Objective 3)

_____ 12. Medicare provisions vary from state to state. (Objectives 3, 5)

_____ 13. Hospitals are required to have a utilization and quality control review program. (Objective 3)

_____ 14. OSHA covers nurses in regard to exposure to toxic chemotherapeutic drugs. (Objective 3)

_____ 15. Most industrialized countries have systems for funding health care that are similar to those in the United States. (Objective 4)

_____ 16. Currently, federal assistance is available for those who do not have private health insurance. (Objective 4)

_____ 17. Budgets for institutions for the retarded and the mentally ill are usually determined at the state level. (Objective 5)

_____ 18. Nurses working for a governmental agency may be prohibited from direct lobbying for funds. (Objective 2)

_____ 19. Running for an office in an organization is considered part of the political process of that organization. (Objective 7)

_____ 20. The techniques of lobbying for a position you favor can be used in a nursing organization. (Objective 7)

Multiple-Choice Questions

_____ 1. One of the reasons the political process is relevant to nurses is that
   a. 35% of the United States population are nurses.
   b. many questions regarding health care are answered through legislation.
   c. nurses are required to report their voting activity.
   d. many nurses serve in state and national legislative positions.
   (Objective 1)

_____ 2. The political process is relevant to nurses because
   a. one's practice as a nurse is controlled by a wide variety of governmental decisions.
   b. many decisions are made within the various nurses' organizations.
   c. health care is costly.
   d. nurses may be drafted in case of war.
   (Objective 1)

_____ 3. The federal agency concerned with planning for the organizations and personnel to provide health care in the community is the
   a. National Institutes of Health.
   b. Food and Drug Administration.
   c. Office of Human Development Services.
   d. Health Resources Administration.
   (Objective 3)

____ 4. Which of the following sources of information about political issues is most likely to be partisan toward a specific political party?

 a. A senator's newsletter

 b. The daily paper

 c. The Federal Registry

 d. A news magazine

 (Objective 2)

____ 5. Which one of the following usually receives the least attention from a legislator?

 a. Mailgrams

 b. Personal letters

 c. Form letters

 d. Telegrams

 (Objective 2)

____ 6. Which of the following results in the most immediate communication of your views to a legislator?

 a. Personal letter

 b. Mailgram

 c. Telephone call

 d. Express mail

 (Objective 2)

____ 7. The cabinet department originally identified as the Department of Health, Education, and Welfare is now known as

 a. the Office of Human Development.

 b. the United States Public Health Service.

 c. the Centers for Disease Control and Prevention.

 d. the Department of Health and Human Services.

 (Objective 3)

_____ 8. To shape the political process, it is most critical that you
   a. be informed.
   b. influence others.
   c. run for office.
   d. write to your senator.
   (Objective 2)

_____ 9. The Public Health Service and the Food and Drug Administration
   are located in which of the following cabinet department?
   a. Health and Human Services
   b. Interior
   c. Health Finance
   d. National Institutes of Health
   (Objective 3)

_____ 10. One of the major concerns with regard to political issues as they
   are related to nursing is
   a. the lack of knowledge on the part of many nurses about the
      political process.
   b. the lack of concern shown by nurses over broad health care
      issues.
   c. the inability of nurses to get political attention.
   d. the fact that so few voters are nurses.
   (Objective 1)

_____ 11. Which of the following is an outcome of the Nurse Education Act?
   a. It provided money for the construction of schools of nursing.
   b. It created an Institute of Nursing in Washington, DC.
   c. It funded the position of Chief Nurse of the United States
      Public Health Service.
   d. It established criteria for being a certified nursing assistant.
   (Objective 30)

_____ 12. The federal act that provided funds for nursing education was known as the
   a.   Social Security Act.
   b.   Comprehensive Health Planning Act.
   c.   Taft-Hartly Act.
   d.   Nurse Education (Training) Act.
   (Objective 3)

_____ 13. One of the effects of the changes in the Nurse Education (Training) Act over the last 5 years has been
   a.   increased financial aid for nursing students.
   b.   decreased financial aid for nursing students.
   c.   increased funding for construction of schools of nursing.
   d.   the channeling of funding away from advanced practice and research and toward basic educational programs.
   (Objective 3)

_____ 14. In 1965, the Social Security Act was amended through Title VIII of the act, which was termed
   a.   Medicare.
   b.   the Maternal-Child Health Act.
   c.   the Health Planning and Utilization Act.
   d.   Medicaid.
   (Objective 3)

_____ 15. Which of the following federal programs provides for chronic renal care?
   a.   Medicare.
   b.   The Health Planning and Utilization Act.
   c.   Medicaid.
   d.   There is no federal assistance for chronic renal dialysis.
   (Objective 3)

____ 16. Medicaid is

    a.   a federal program administered by the participating individual states.

    b.   a federal program administered by the United States Health Department.

    c.   a state program entirely financed and directed by states.

    d.   a federal program administered by local governmental agencies.

(Objectives 3)

____ 17. The amount of money available under any federal legislative act depends on

    a.   the appropriated amount only.

    b.   the authorized amount only.

    c.   the agency's spending decisions.

    d.   all of the above.

(Objective 3)

____ 18. The act that governs working conditions for nurses handling toxic chemotherapeutic agents is the

    a.   Maternal-Child Health Act.

    b.   OSHA.

    C.   Professional Standards Review Act.

    d.   Health Planning and Resources Development Act.

(Objective 3)

____ 19. Which of the following statements accurately expresses the current states of health planning and resources development?

    a.   Federal support is available for local areas willing to match funds.

    b.   Federal support is available without the need for matching funds locally.

    c.   Federal support takes the form of advisers who work with local agencies.

    d.   There is no federal support for health planning and resources development.

(Objective 3)

____ 20. What major problem is creating support for some type of govern-
ment-sponsored health care plan?
   a.   The high cost of renal dialysis
   b.   The increasing elderly population
   c.   Uncompensated care
   d.   Pressure for new technology
   (Objective 4)

____ 21. To affect the funding of health care for the state prison system, one
would need to lobby
   a.   the Department of Health and Human Services
   b.   the congressional representative for one's district.
   c.   prison administrative officials.
   d.   the budget committee for one's state legislature.
   (Objective 5)

____ 22. To affect funding for the local health department, one would need
to lobby
   a.   the United States Public Health Service.
   b.   the congressional representative for one's district.
   c.   administrative officials of the public health department.
   d.   the county/city council.
   (Objective 6)

____ 23. Whether nurse practitioners are allowed to practice is determined
at the
   a.   federal level.
   b.   state level.
   c.   local level.
   d.   All of the above
   (Objective 6)

11 | Beginning Your Career as a Nurse

Purpose

This chapter helps the student to look toward employment as a nurse. Social changes affecting the new graduate, the various views of competency, and expectations of employers are discussed to assist students as they plan their own entry into the work force. Suggestions for coping with expectations of others and for setting personal career goals are provided. Concrete directions are given for applying for a position, writing a resume, and responding to an interview. The discussion of reality shock burnout is designed to help the student prepare for these possibilities and approach them constructively.

Objectives

1. *Discuss the historical development of employment roles for nurses.*

2. *Describe a variety of employment opportunities available to nurses today.*

3. *Explain the common competencies by the new graduate as outlined by the job analysis study.*

4. *Analyze the eight common expectations employers have of new graduates and relate them to your own background and education.*

5. *Develop a list of your personal short- and long-term career goals.*

6. *Describe how you plan to maintain your competence in nursing.*

7. *Create a personal resumé; sample letters of application, follow-up, and resignation; and a plan for your personal responses in an employment interview that can be used when you seek employment.*

8. *Explore strategies that you might personally use to prevent or alleviate reality shock.*

9. *Analyze your own values and life situation in relationship to your personal potential for burnout.*

10. *Discuss two areas of concern relative to sex discrimination in nursing.*

11. *Identify ways that you act to protect the health of both yourself and others in the nursing workplace.*

Key Terms

burnout	expert
community health care	long-term care
comparable worth	novice
competency	reality shock
criticality	resumé
discrimination	stereotype

Situations to Foster Critical Thinking

1. Analyze your own background and identify your strengths and weaknesses. Develop an approach to presenting your strengths to a prospective employer and create a plan for your own growth.

2. In your clinical practice setting, identify the skills that nurses are currently using. Compare this with the common expectations outlined in the text and with what you know about other settings in your community.

3. Analyze the concept of reality shock and evaluate your own potential for experiencing this phenomenon. Do you believe that this is a problem to be avoided or a naturally occurring professional development phenomenon?

4. Set a short term career goal and long-term career goal. Identify the steps you will need to take to reach those goals.

5. There are few job opportunities for newly licensed registered nurses in your community. To conduct a successful job search, you will need to plan carefully. First, identify the various settings that might employ a new graduate in your community. Then outline the key skills and abilities you believe would be needed in each setting. Lastly, evaluate yourself in relationship to these key skills and abilities.

6. Develop a comprehensive list of questions that you believe might be asked in an employment interview for a registered nurse in your community. Plan personal answers to these questions.

Discussion/Essay Questions

1. Identify a major change in the way health care is delivered and how this has affected the abilities of the new graduate. (Objective 1)

2. Identify a major change in the way nursing education is conducted and how this has affected the abilities of the new graduate. (Objective 1)

3. How has technology affected the role of the new graduate in nursing? (Objective 1)

4. Define competency as it applies to nursing and discuss how this will affect your practice as a beginning nurse. (Objective 3)

5. Compare the areas of competence that are of concern to employers with the nursing education you have received and evaluate yourself in relationship to these areas. (Objective 4)

6. Identify three of the consistent expectations that employers have of new graduates and discuss how you can act to meet those expectations. (Objective 4)

7. Identify one common area in which employers expect competence and discuss how you feel prepared to function in that area. (Objective 4)

8. Do you feel prepared to meet employers' expectations in regard to theoretical knowledge and use of the nursing process? Explain your answer. (Objective 4)

9. Two areas in which employers' expectations differ widely were mentioned. What is the situation in your geographical area in regard to these expectations? (Objective 4)

10. What avenues are open to you to make yourself better prepared to meet employers' expectations? How might you go about using these? (Objective 6)

11. Briefly sketch a description of what you expect to be doing professionally five, ten, and twenty years after graduation. (Objective 5)

12. What should you include in a letter of application? (Objective 7)

13. What should you include in a resume? (Objective 7)

14. What do you see as your greatest assets in an interview? Your greatest liabilities? (Objective 7)

15. Discuss how you might use an interview follow-up letter to increase your chances of obtaining a position you desire. (Objective 7)

16. Discuss ways in which you might tactfully indicate in a letter of resignation that you were leaving because the setting did not provide an opportunity for staff nurses to be involved in decision-making about the delivery of nursing care. (Objective 7)

17. Define burnout and describe factors in nursing employment situations that might contribute to burnout. (Objective 9)

18. Identify specific actions you might take on your own behalf that could prevent reality shock. (Objective 8)

19. Discuss whether sex discrimination has affected the men enrolled in your nursing program. (Objective 10)

20. Identify actions that nurses could take to eliminate sex discrimination in nursing. (Objective 10)

Fill-In-The-Blank Questions

1. The number of nurses employed outside of the hospital setting today is _____ than the past. (Objective 2)

2. The organization that defined competency as "a combination of demonstrated cognitive, affected, and/or psychomotor capabilities derived from the activities of the associate degree nurse in the various roles in the practice setting" was the _____ _____. (Objective 3)

3. The groups for which the NLN provided competency statements are __ _____ , and _____. (Objective 3)

4. Three consistent expectations that employers have of new graduates are _____, _____, and _____. (Objective 4)

5. Reality shock is defined as _____. (Objective 8)

6. Individuals who will attest to your abilities as an employee are termed _____. (Objective 7)

7. _____ are more likely to be the object of sex discrimination in nursing. (Objective 10)

8. A letter of resignation is usually sent _____ weeks before you will leave employment. (Objective 7)

True-False Questions

_____ 1. In the early part of the 20th century, most nurses were employed by hospitals. (Objective 1)

_____ 2. The 1930s saw a change in nursing in that nurses were no longer expected to be "on duty" for an entire 24-hour period. (Objective 1)

_____ 3. One change in nursing created by World War II was the employment of married nurses. (Objective 1)

_____ 4. In the 1940s, most graduates of hospital schools of nursing were employed by the hospitals in which they received their education. (Objective 1)

_____ 5. Competency refers to the ability to perform as expected. (Objective 3)

_____ 6. Changes in nursing education in the last 20 years have resulted in not every student having an opportunity to perform every skill. (Objective 3)

_____ 7. Employers are generally concerned with the new nurse's ability to use technical skills. (Objective 4)

___ 8. Employers generally expect that they will have to teach the nursing process to new nurses. (Objective 4)

___ 9. Employers generally expect new nurses to know their own strengths and weaknesses and to ask for help. (Objective 4)

___ 10. Employers generally do not expect that new nurses will understand the demands of record-keeping. (Objective 4)

___ 11. There are wide differences in the degree of technical skill that employers expect of new nurses. (Objective 5)

___ 12. There is general agreement about the speed at which new nurses are expected to function. (Objective 4)

___ 13. Reality shock refers to feelings that result from encountering a more complex and difficult work situation than expected and feeling powerless to affect the situation. (Objective 8)

___ 14. An externship is a program to help nursing students become more familiar and comfortable with the employment setting while they are still students. (Objective 8)

___ 15. For the new graduate, personal career goals should focus on the short-term only. (Objective 5)

___ 16. A letter of application should include an overview of the applicant's qualifications for the position being sought. (Objective 7)

___ 17. A resumé should include reference to special honors or recognition received while a nursing student. (Objective 7)

___ 18. A resumé should include offices held in social organizations. (Objective 7)

___ 19. It is inappropriate to ask questions regarding salary and benefits in an interview. (Objective 7)

___ 20. It is appropriate to ask questions regarding policies and procedures during an interview. (Objective 7)

___ 21. After an interview, you should wait for the employer to contact you. (Objective 7)

___ 22. An interview follow-up letter includes a reference to any agreements or commitments made by the employer during the interview. (Objective 7)

___ 23. If you have been unhappy in a job, the letter of resignation is the best place to inform your employer of your grievances. (Objective 7)

___ 24. A formal letter of resignation is necessary only if you have a management position. (Objective 7)

_____ 25. A letter of resignation is often sent to more than one person in the organization. (Objective 7)

_____ 26. Burnout is more likely to happen in units that have inadequate staffing. (Objective 9)

Multiple-Choice Questions

_____ 1. Which of the following has historically been the setting in which most new graduates were employed?

a. Hospital

b. Health-related businesses

c. Outpatient setting

d. Community nursing agency

(Objective 1)

_____ 2. Which of the following has decreased the new graduate's ability to perform according to the hospital's procedures?

a. New graduates do not learn procedures anymore.

b. Individuals are not necessarily employed in institutions where they had education experiences.

c. Most new nurses have less education than previously.

d. The focus of nursing education is on outpatient care, not hospital care.

(Objective 3)

_____ 3. Recently nursing organizations and groups have looked at various educational paths to nursing education to define what those who follow each should be able to do. These abilities have been termed

a. outcome behaviors.

b. competencies.

c. levels of performance.

d. skills

(Objective 3)

___ 4. Employers want to be sure that
   a. new graduates will possess the necessary theoretical background for basic patient care and decision-making.
   b. new graduates will function efficiently within one week of assuming a new position.
   c. new graduates will not need a lot of supervision after the first month.
   d. new graduates will understand hospital policies.
   (Objective 4)

___ 5. Which of the following is an expectation that employers consistently have of new employees?
   a. That they perform all technical skills without assistance
   b. That they are comfortable with hospital policy
   c. That they will recognize their own abilities and limitations
   d. That they will be able to assume charge of the unit in six months
   (Objective 4)

___ 6. What is expected of the new graduate in regard to record-keeping?
   a. Records should be completed independently.
   b. The new graduate will not be responsible for records is expected.
   c. The ability to use computerized records is expected.
   d. The new graduate must know what must be recorded.
   (Objective 4)

___ 7. Most employers of new graduates expect that the new graduate will
   a. be skilled in carrying out procedures.
   b. be efficient in carrying out responsibilities.
   c. be able to use the nursing process effectively.
   d. be proficient in the charting system in use.
   (Objective 4)

____ 8. In which of the following may expectations of the new graduate vary widely?

    a.   In different facilities and in different geographical areas

    b.   From one graduate of the program to another

    c.   From one class to another

    d.   Within the same geographical area

    (Objective 4)

____ 9. Which of the following is the least effective method of coping with expectations of the employer?

    a.   Review your own abilities before graduation and seek experiences.

    b.   Look for employment only in a facility where you practiced as a student.

    c.   Seek an employer with an orientation program that matches your needs.

    d.   Start a support group with other new graduates.

    (Objective 8)

____ 10. In setting your personal goals, a recommended first step is to

    a.   review the clinical evaluation done while you were a student.

    b.   ask your friends what they think you would do the best.

    c.   do a thorough self-assessment.

    d.   determine which areas of the hospital need your help the most.

    (Objective 5)

____ 11. What is the best length for a resume for a new graduate?

    a.   One page

    b.   Two pages

    c.   Three pages

    d.   Four pages

    (Objective 7)

_____ 12. In preparing for an interview, you should
   a. outline questions you will want to ask.
   b. be as casual as possible.
   c. consider canceling the interview and rescheduling later if are too nervous.
   d. purchase a new suit so you will look professional.
   (Objective 7)

_____ 13. Which of the following is the most critical in an interview?
   a. Be neat and well groomed
   b. Have a good understanding of the philosophy of the hospital
   c. Do not act nervous
   d. Limit comments to the answers to questions posed by the interviewer
   (Objective 7)

_____ 14. Which of the following is essential to presenting yourself effectively in an interview for a beginning nursing position?
   a. Have your hair done professionally
   b. Take a class on interviewing techniques
   c. Purchase new "businesslike" clothing
   d. Reflect on your personal philosophy of nursing
   (Objective 7)

_____ 15. A major purpose of an interview follow-up letter is to
   a. add information you forgot to give in your interview.
   b. ask additional questions about the organization.
   c. restate any agreements that were reached.
   d. review important points you made during the interview.
   (Objective 7)

_____ 16. A letter of resignation should be directed to
   a. the hospital administrator.
   b. the nursing administrator.
   c. the personnel department.
   d. your shift charge nurse.
   (Objective 7)

_____ 17. The situation in which the new graduate becomes frustrated because it may seem impossible to deliver quality care under the constraints in force is known as

    a. disassociation.

    b. reality shock.

    c. displacement.

    d. burnout.

    (Objective 8)

_____ 18. A program designed to provide a planned, organized transition period in which the new graduate participates in classes, seminars, and rotations to various units of the hospital is known as

    a. on-the-job training.

    b. orientation.

    c. externship.

    d. internship.

    (Objective 8)

_____ 19. Which of the following is a personal strategy that might effectively combat burnout without jeopardizing your career?

    a. Decrease your physical exercise to conserve energy

    b. Plan for a group of nurses to share concerns

    c. Stay no longer than one year in a position

    d. Take extra vitamins

    (Objective 8)

_____ 20. An area of recent economic concern in nursing is

    a. comparable worth.

    b. nepotism.

    c. civil rights.

    d. shift differentials.

    (Objective 10)

_____ 21. An employment area in nursing that has sometimes been discriminatory toward men in nursing is
   a. long-term care.
   b. obstetrics.
   c. pediatrics.
   d. surgery.
   (Objective 13)

_____ 22. Employers may be required to provide employees who have significant risk with immunization for
   a. AIDS.
   b. tetanus.
   c. hepatitis B.
   d. tuberculosis.
   (Objective 14)

_____ 23. Which of the following work-related hazards is present in almost every area of nursing?
   a. Anesthetic gases
   b. AIDS
   c. Chemotherapeutic agents
   d. Toxic chemicals
   (Objective 14)

12 | Understanding Nursing Employment Settings

Purpose

The majority of new graduates begin their lives as registered nurses working for an organization or agency that provides health care services. To help them function more effectively in those settings, this chapter presents basic information about hospitals, nursing homes, and community agencies. Information on the classification and governance of agencies and on the roles of the various groups (such as board, administration, and medical staff) has been included. The mechanisms for functioning within an organizational framework are explored. The various ways in which the delivery of nursing care is organized and how nurses relate to those structures are discussed.

Objectives

1. *Describe the various settings in which newly registered nurses may begin practice.*

2. *Describe the three general classifications of health care agencies.*

3. *Discuss the early development of hospitals and nursing homes and the factors affecting that development.*

4. *Describe the health care delivery provided in ambulatory care settings and community agencies.*

5. *Explain the roles of the governing board, the administrator, the medical staff, and the nursing administrator in a health care agency.*

6. *Outline the use of clinical ladders as opportunities for nurses.*

7. *Discuss the purposes of a mission statement, policies and procedures, standards of care, and quality improvement processes in a health care agency.*

8. *Define terms used in describing organizational structure including channels of communication, chain of command, centralized structure, decentralized structure, and organizational chart.*

9. *Compare the various patterns of nursing care delivery and how they are integrated into different care environments.*

Key Terms

acute care hospitals

care pathways

case manager

case method of care delivery

centralized structure

chain of command

channels of communication

clinical ladder

community mental health
centers

continuous quality
improvement (CQI)

decentralized structure

functional care

job description

long-term care facility

mission statement

nursing home

nonprofit

organizational chart

organizational hierarchy

organizational structure

patterns of care delivery

policy

primary nursing

procedure

protocol

proprietary agency

quality improvement

subacute care

team nursing

tertiary care hospital

total quality management
(TQM)

transitional care

Situations to Foster Critical Thinking

1. The nursing home in which you are employed is instituting a continuous quality improvement program. What factors in this program will affect your work as a registered nurse? What questions do you need to ask to understand the impact of this particular program on expectations of you? Of whom will you ask these questions?

2. You are employed in an acute care hospital and have been informed that the pattern of care delivery is to be changed from primary nursing to a modular approach to care in which each module will have one registered nurse and two other care providers. These two additional care providers may be licensed practical nurses, nursing students, or nursing assistants. What are the skills you will need in this new pattern of care delivery that you did not need in the original pattern? What concerns will you have about this new pattern of care delivery? What questions do you need to ask to plan for the transition? What are the benefits and the drawbacks to this new pattern?

3. You have identified that the system for recording medication administration in the subacute care unit where you work requires that p.r.n. medications be recorded in three different places and that frequently one of these is omitted by the nurses. This causes confusion and you find yourself spending excessive time checking and double-checking. How might you seek to change this procedure? Consider the lines of authority and accountability and roles of various individuals as you plan. What information do you need before you take any action?

4. You work for a home health agency providing care for eight-hour shifts to high acuity children. You have been assigned to a new client who requires ventilator management. You have never cared for such a child in the past. How would you respond to your supervisor in regard to this assignment? What resources in the agency might be available to assist you?

Discussion/Essay Questions

1. Discuss how the development of hospitals has been affected by the needs and pressures of society. (Objective 3)

2. Discuss how their origin as almshouses has affected the development of hospitals in the United States. (Objective 3)

3. Describe how technology has affected the development of the modern hospital in the United States. (Objective 3)

4. Differentiate between proprietary and nonprofit health care agencies. (Objective 2)

5. Discuss three ways in which health care agencies are classified. (Objective 2)

6. Identify how the board of trustees (or governors) at a local health care agency is chosen. Discuss how this process might affect the goals and priorities of the agency. (Objective 3)

7. Examine the organizational chart of a local health care agency. What is the title of highest-level administrator, and who reports to that individual? (Objective 8)

8. How do physicians gain the privilege of practicing at a hospital? (Objective 5)

9. Identify all of the agencies in your community that hire newly licensed registered nurses. (Objective 1)

10. What is the title of the highest-level nursing administrator in your local hospital, and who reports to that individual? (Objective 8)

11. Identify the mission statement or statement of purpose and philosophy of a local health care agency. Analyze how this statement affects the type of services offered. (Objective 7)

12. Make a chart of the reporting relationships on a unit of the hospital where you have practiced as a student. Be sure to include all positions found on that unit. (Objective 8)

13. Is the hospital where you had your most recent clinical experience designed with a tall organizational structure or a flat one? Why do you believe this? (Objective 8)

14. What health care agencies in your community are public/governmental? (Objective 2)

15. How would the presence or absence of a quality improvement program in a hospital affect your functioning as a beginning staff nurse in that setting? (Objective 7)

16. Compare and contrast primary, team, and functional nursing. (Objective 9)

17. Analyze the structure for delivering nursing care in the hospital where you had your most recent experience. Which form does it most nearly resemble and what are the differences, if any? (Objective 9)

18. Identify ways in which a clinical ladder might serve to enhance your personal satisfaction with nursing. (Objective 6)

Fill-In-The-Blank Questions

1. The average length of stay in an acute care hospital is usually measured in _____. (Objective 2)

2. The first hospital in the United States was in the state of _____. (Objective 3)

3. Dorothea Dix is famous for her campaigns to reform treatment for the _____. (Objective 3)

4. A facility is considered a short-stay facility if the average stay is less than _____ days. (Objective 2)

5. Policy for a hospital is set by the _____. (Objective 5)

6. The _____ is responsible for ensuring that the activities of the hospital are consistent with the goals and policies established by the board. (Objective 5)

7. The group that has responsibility for evaluating medical care in a hospital is the _____. (Objective 5)

8. The person who holds the highest nursing position in a hospital is commonly termed the _____. (Objective 5)

9. The statement that indicates the broad aims of a hospital is called its __ _____. (Objective 7)

10. An organization in which each management person has many individuals reporting to her or him is said to have a _____ span of control. (Objective 8)

11. An organization with many levels of management is said to have ____ _____ structure. (Objective 8)

12. Conferences among those who are providing care to a group of patients are essential to the functioning of _____ nursing. (Objective 9)

13. In _____ nursing, one nurse has 24-hour responsibility for planning care for an individual patient. (Objective 9)

14. A structure in which a nurse may remain in patient care and still receive advancement in position and salary is called a _____. (Objective 6)

True-False Questions

_____ 1. In the United States, the earliest institutions to care for those with communicable diseases were called pesthouses. (Objective 2)

_____ 2. Early hospitals in the United States enforced strict standards of cleanliness. (Objective 2)

_____ 3. X-rays and laboratory tests were first used in hospitals in the 20th century. (Objective 2)

_____ 4. Nursing contributed to the growth of hospitals through increased attention to cleanliness and nutrition. (Objective 2)

_____ 5. A nonprofit health care agency is one that provides charity care and expects to lose money. (Objective 2)

_____ 6. A proprietary agency is investor owned. (Objective 2)

_____ 7. A board of governors is always elected by the community. (Objective 5)

_____ 8. The hospital administrator must be knowledgeable in business management. (Objective 5)

_____ 9. All individuals who admit and treat patients at a hospital must be admitted to the medical staff. (Objective 5)

_____ 10. If a physician is identified as providing poor care, it is the responsibility of the hospital administrator to remove that physician from the staff of the hospital. (Objective 5)

_____ 11. Nursing is usually the largest single health care occupation in a hospital. (Objective 5)

_____ 12. The highest-level nursing position in a hospital is always vice-president. (Objective 5)

_____ 13. A mission statement usually identifies the general purposes of the organization. (Objective 7)

_____ 14. When using a chain of command correctly, you would report a problem to your immediate supervisor before reporting it to the director of nursing. (Objective 8)

_____ 15. In a flat organizational structure, the individual usually has a narrow span of control. (Objective 8)

_____ 16. Quality improvement is aimed at identifying poor practice in health care. (Objective 7)

_____ 17. In a total patient care method of assignment, the nurse has responsibility for planning and supervising the individual patient's care for 24 hours a day. (Objective 9)

_____ 18. All case managers are registered nurses with a baccalaureate degree. (Objective 9)

_____ 19. All case managers follow patients from before admission, throughout hospitalization, and until they are discharged from home care. (Objective 9)

_____ 20. A clinical ladder is designed to allow nurses to remain in patient care while being promoted in level and salary. (Objective 6)

Multiple-Choice Questions

_____ 1. Dorothea Dix campaigned for humane treatment of
   a. children with disabilities.
   b. pregnant women.
   c. the mentally ill.
   d. those with communicable diseases.
   (Objective 3)

_____ 2. Hospitals that are operated to provide a return on investment for stockholders are called
   a. nonprofit.
   b. proprietary.
   c. public.
   d. voluntary.
   (Objective 2)

_____ 3. The ultimate fiscal responsibility for a hospital resides with the
   a. administrator.
   b. board of trustees.
   c. medical staff.
   d. government.
   (Objective 4)

_____ 4. Responsibility for day-to-day financial management of a hospital lies with the
   a. administrator.
   b. board of trustees.
   c. medical staff.
   d. government.
   (Objective 5)

_____ 5. Responsibility for monitoring the quality of medical care in a hospital lies with the
   a. administrator.
   b. board of trustees.
   c. medical staff.
   d. government.
   (Objective 5)

_____ 6. Responsibility for direction of nursing services in a hospital usually rests with the
   a. administrator.
   b. director of nursing.
   c. medical staff.
   d. nursing staff.
   (Objective 5)

_____ 7. The broad goals of a hospital are usually found in its
   a. articles of incorporation.
   b. mission statement.
   c. policy manual.
   d. procedure manual.
   (Objective 7)

____ 8. The plan that describes reporting relationships in an organization is called the
   a. chain of command.
   b. channel of communication.
   c. clinical ladder.
   d. span of control.
   (Objective 8)

____ 9. A program designed to move an agency toward upgrading consumer service rather than merely meeting current standards is titled
   a. diagnosis-related groups.
   b. preferred provider organization.
   c. quality assurance.
   d. quality improvement.
   (Objective 7)

____ 10. In which pattern of care delivery is each person responsible for specific tasks?
   a. Functional nursing
   b. Primary nursing
   c. Team nursing
   d. Total patient care
   (Objective 9)

____ 11. A plan that allows the staff nurse to be promoted without leaving patient care is called a
   a. career pathway.
   b. clinical ladder.
   c. proprietary technique.
   d. support system.
   (Objective 6)

13 | Organizations for and About Nursing

Purpose

Many organizations are related to the nursing profession. These organizations affect the profession and can provide support to the individual nurse in numerous ways. This chapter is directed toward helping the student understand these organizations, their purposes and activities, and how they relate to one another. It is hoped that this information will provide direction as the student decides which organizations to join as a practicing nurse.

Objectives

1. Discuss reasons for the existence of the large number of nursing organizations.

2. Identify the purposes of the major structural units of the American Nurses Association (ANA) and how they carry out the activities and programs of the ANA.

3. Explain the purposes of the International Council of Nursing, the American Nurses Foundation, and the American Academy of Nursing.

4. Identify the major structural units of the National League for Nursing (NLN) and how these support its purposes, programs, and activities.

5. Differentiate the criteria for membership in the NLN and the ANA.

6. Outline the activities of the National Student Nurses' Association (NSNA).

7. Describe the organizations representing licensed practical nurses.

8. Discuss the major purpose of each specialized organization presented in the chapter.

Key Terms

accreditation
American Academy of Nursing
American Nurses Association
American Nurses Foundation
consultation
continuing education
evaluation and testing

International Council of
Nurses

lobbying

membership

National Council of State
Boards of Nursing

National Federation of
Licensed Practical
Nurses

National League for Nursing

National Student Nurses'
Association

organizational structure

specialty organizations

research

Situations to Foster Critical Thinking

1. You and another new graduate are discussing nursing organizations. She has asked whether you would join the specialty organization or the ANA. Identify your personal viewpoint and the rationale supporting your decision.

2. Some members of the nursing staff at the hospital where you work are putting together a proposal to support two nurses to attend a national convention of the ANA. Would you support this proposal? Outline the rationale underlying your position. Identify the strongest arguments in opposition to your position.

3. A proposal is before a specialty organization to which you belong to join its certification program with the ANA Credentialing Center. Identify the benefits and the drawbacks for the specialty organization in losing its certification program.

4. Identify whether your nursing program is accredited by the NLN. What benefits are there in attending a nursing education program that is nationally accredited? Which of these benefits is of value to you and why?

Discussion/Essay Questions

1. Why are there so many different nursing organizations? (Objective 1)

2. What problems for nursing might the proliferation of organizations cause? (Objective 1)

3. What is the major function of the Board of Directors of the ANA? (Objective 2)

4. What is the role of the ANA in relationship to actions of the federal government? (Objective 2)

5. What services does the ANA provide that benefit the individual members? (Objective 2)

6. Outline the major areas that the NSNA addresses. (Objective 6)
7. What is the general purpose of the NLN? (Objective 4)
8. Give your views on why the NLN allows nonnurses as members. What benefits and what problems does this create for the organization? (Objective 4)
9. If two levels of nursing, technical and professional, become a standard, what do you believe the membership requirements for the ANA should be, and why? (Objective 2)
10. What is the role of the NLN in relationship to community health agencies? (Objective 4)
11. What is the NLN accreditation? Do you believe it is of value to a nursing program? Explain your answer. (Objective 4)

Fill-In-The-Blank Questions

1. The decision to join nursing organizations is usually a (an) _____ as well as a philosophical one. (Objective 1).
2. The Constituent Assembly includes presidents and executive directors of _____. (Objective 2)
3. *Facts About Nursing*, a report of basic statistical information, is published by the _____. (Objective 4)
4. "Breakthrough into Nursing" is a project of the NSNA for the purpose of _____. (Objective 6)
5. The prime purpose of the NLN is to _____. (Objective 4)
6. In addition to nurses, _____ are eligible for membership in the NLN. (Objective 4)
7. The organization that provides for accreditation of nursing programs is the _____. (Objective 4)
8. The organization that provides for accreditation of agencies offering home health service is the _____. (Objective 4)
9. Is national accreditation of nursing programs voluntary or required? _____ (Objective 4)
10. The organization that recognizes individual nurses who have demonstrated outstanding scholarship and leadership for the profession is the _____. (Objective 3)
11. The letters FAAN stand for _____. (Objective 3)
12. The organization formed by the ANA as a political action arm is _____ _____. (Objective 2)

True-False Questions

_____ 1. Different nursing organizations have been formed to meet different needs identified in the profession. (Objective 1)

_____ 2. The House of Delegates of the ANA sets policy for the organization. (Objective 2)

_____ 3. The Board of Directors of the ANA sets policy for the organization. (Objective 2)

_____ 4. The ANA accredits schools of nursing. (Objectives 2, 4)

_____ 5. The ANA financially supports the NSNA. (Objective 6)

_____ 6. The ANA speaks for the profession of nursing to the general public. (Objective 2)

_____ 7. The NSNA is supporting the recruitment and retention of minorities in the field of nursing. (Objective 6)

_____ 8. The NSNA is a completely independent organization. (Objective 6)

_____ 9. The NLN promotes quality nursing care in all settings. (Objective 4)

_____ 10. Both organizations and individuals may join the NLN. (Objective 4)

_____ 11. Individual nurses may join the ANA directly. (Objective 2)

_____ 12. The NLN provides national accreditation for schools of nursing. (Objective 4)

_____ 13. The NLN does not involve itself in politics. (Objective 4)

_____ 14. National accreditation is required for graduates of a program to receive interstate endorsement of their licenses. (Objective 4)

_____ 15. Most specialty organizations provide continuing education for their members.

_____ 16. FAAN stands for Fellow of the American Academy of Nursing. (Objective 3)

_____ 17. The American Nurses Foundation supports research in nursing. (Objective 3)

_____ 18. The National Council of State Boards of Nursing sets licensing requirements. (Objective 8)

Multiple-Choice Questions

_____ 1. A serious concern raised by the existence of so many organizations in the field of nursing is
   a. the restrictions on membership.
   b. the overlapping of function and interrelationships.
   c. which one is the best organization.
   d. which one is government approved.
   (Objective 1)

_____ 2. The major nursing organization that started with a meeting of nursing leaders at the World's Fair in Chicago in 1890 is the
   a. NLN.
   b. Black Nurses Association.
   c. ANA.
   d. American College of Nurse Midwives.
   (Objective 2)

_____ 3. The nursing organization that has as one of its major concerns the economic welfare of nurses is the
   a. NLN.
   b. AWHONN.
   c. Association of Operating Room Nurses.
   d. ANA.
   (Objective 2)

_____ 4. The NSNA is
   a. a branch of the ANA.
   b. a branch of the NLN.
   c. supported by the American Hospital Association.
   d. a fully independent organization.
   (Objective 6)

____ 5. The NLN supports quality nursing care through

    a. assisting nurses who are striving for better economic conditions.

    b. accrediting home health care agencies.

    c. giving scholarships to outstanding students in nursing.

    d. providing grants for nursing research.

    (Objective 4)

____ 6. The nursing organization whose membership is limited to registered nurses is

    a. the NLN.

    b. NAACOG.

    c. the Association of Operating Room Nurses.

    d. the ANA.

    (Objective 2)

____ 7. The nursing organization that accredits nursing education programs is the

    a. NLN.

    b. NSNA.

    c. ANA.

    d. American Association of Colleges of Nursing (AACN).

    (Objective 4)

____ 8. The purpose of accreditation is to

    a. facilitate interstate movement of nurses.

    b. assist with licensure.

    c. support excellence in curriculum.

    d. help faculty know what should be taught.

    (Objective 4)

_____ 9. The nursing organization to which new members are elected by those currently in the organization is the

    a. NLN.

    b. American Academy of Nursing.

    c. ANA.

    d. American College of Nurse Midwives.

    (Objective 3)

_____ 10. The nursing organization that meets once every four years is the

    a. International Council of Nurses.

    b. National Nursing Ethics Organization.

    c. Federation of Nurse Practitioners.

    d. ANA.

    (Objective 3)

_____ 11. The delegates to the convention of the ANA are responsible for

    a. confirming all appointments to offices.

    b. determining the methods to be used to achieve goals.

    c. establishing the budget for the ANA.

    d. making policies to guide the organization.

    (Objective 2)

_____ 12. The Board of Directors of the ANA is responsible for

    a. electing all officers.

    b. making policies.

    c. hiring the executive director.

    d. selecting representatives for the Constituent Assembly.

    (Objective 2)

_____ 13. The Student Bill of Rights for nursing was developed by the

    a. ANA

    b. National Council of State Boards.

    c. NLN.

    d. NSNA.

    (Objective 6)

____ 14. Which of the following organizations is focused on nursing research?

   a.   ANA

   b.   American Nurses Foundation

   c.   NLN

   d.   NSNA

   (Objective 3)

Answer Key

Chapter 1 - Nursing as a Developing Profession

Fill-In-The-Blank Questions

1. diagnosis; treatment
2. technological
3. Virginia Henderson
4. ANA; National Council of State Boards of Nursing
5. collegiate settings
6. Code for Nurses
7. Egypt
8. disease prevention
9. yin; yang
10. Greek
11. folk; religious; servant
12. deaconesses
13. St. Macella, Fabioloa, and St. Paula
14. change in the role of women
15. Reformation
16. Florence Nightingale
17. Pennsylvania Hospital
18. Clara Barton
19. New England Hospital for Women and Children
20. newspapers; news magazines
21. Dorothea Dix
22. Harriet Tubman, Susie Taylor, and Sjourner Truth
23. nursing eduction
24. Winslow-Goldmark Report
25. Mildred Montag
26. the roles of nurses in the delivery of health care educational patterns that would encourage capable individuals to choose nursing, and programs that would facilitate educational mobility
27. pin
28. pediatric; psychiatric
29. religion
30. 21

True-False Questions

1. F
2. T
3. T
4. F
5. T
6. T
7. T
8. F
9. T
10. F
11. F
12. T

13.	F
14.	T
15.	F
16.	F
17.	T
18.	T
19.	T
20.	T

Matching Questions

A.
1. e
2. f
3. a
4. b
5. c
6. d

B.
1. d
2. e
3. a
4. c
5. f
6. b

Multiple Choice Questions

1. a
2. a
3. b
4. c
5. b
6. c
7. c
8. b
9. d
10. a

11. c
12. c
13. b
14. c
15. d
16. a
17. c
18. a
19. c
20. a
21. d
22. c
23. a
24. d
25. c
26. a
27. a
28. c
29. b
30. c

Chapter 2 - Educational Preparation for Nursing

Fill-In-The-Blank Questions

1. Omnibus Budget Reconciliation Act
2. registered nurse; licensed practical (vocational) nurse
3. varies from state to state
4. YWCA
5. 9; 1
6. vocational
7. 1940s
8. vocational-technical schools and community colleges

9. hospital-based diploma; bac-calaureate; two-year associate degree
10. hospital-based diploma
11. affiliation
12. immediately assume the re-sponsibilities of a staff position

13. expense
14. the University of Minnesota
15. upper-division major in nurs-ing
16. 4-year colleges; universities
17. baccalaureate degree
18. 1952
19. Mildred Montag
20. junior and community colleges
21. registered nurse baccalaureate program
22. master's
23. internships
24. internships; orientation pro-grams; residencies
25. help prepare individuals for roles of increased breadth and scope
26. articulated
27. ladder
28. meetings or conventions
29. continuing education
30. volunatary; mandatory

True-False Questions

1. F
2. T
3. T

4. F
5. T
6. F
7. T
8. T
9. F
10. T
11. T
12. F
13. F
14. F
15. T
16. F
17. T
18. T
19. F
20. T

Matching Questions

A.
1. d
2. f
3. c
4. b
5. e

6. a

B.
1. e
2. b
3. d
4. c
5. a

Multiple-Choice Questions

1. c

2. c
3. d
4. a
5. b
6. b
7. b
8. d
9. c
10. c
11. d
12. c
13. a
14. d
15. d
16. b
17. b
18. d
19. b
20. c
21. c
22. d
23. c
24. c
25. c
26. b
27. a
28. a
29. d
30. b

Chapter 3 - Perspectives on Nursing Education

Fill-In-The-Blank Questions

1. Nursing for the Future
2. social; technical; political; financial
3. National League for Nursing
4. institutions of higher education
5. baccalaureate degree in nursing
6. associate degree in nursing
7. North Dakota
8. scope of practice
9. grandfather
10. titling; grandfather clause
11. interstate endorsement
12. compentencies
13. computers
14. educational mobility
15. community-based
16. Nurse Training Act
17. adaptation
18. systems
19. Martha Rogers
20. self-care
21. Virginia Henderson
22. interpersonal relationship

True-False Questions

1. T
2. T
3. F
4. T
5. T
6. F
7. F
8. T
9. T
10. F

11. T
12. F
13. T
14. F
15. T
16. T
17. T
18. F
19. F
20. F
21. T
22. T
23. F
24. F
25. F

Matching Questions

A.
1. b
2. d
3. e
4. a
5. c

B.
1. c
2. a
3. e
4. b
5. d

C.
1. c
2. a
3. e
4. b
5. d

Multiple-Choice Questions

1. d
2. a
3. b
4. a
5. c
6. d
7. b
8. a
9. a
10. b
11. c
12. b
13. d
14. a
15. a
16. c
17. b
18. d
19. a
20. b
21. d
22. d
23. a
24. c
25. c
26. a
27. a
28. d
29. a
30. c
31. d
32. d
33. c

Chapter 4 - Credentials for Health Care Providers

Fill-In-The-Blank

1. protect the public; support professionals
2. state; professional organization
3. Nurses Associated Alumnae of the United States and Canada later known as the American Nurses Association (ANA)
4. Permissive
5. New York
6. continuing education
7. American Nurses Association
8. baccalaureate
9. American Nurses Association and its precursor
10. (Any three) performing services for compensation; necessity for specialized knowledge base; use of nursing process; components of nursing practice; execution of the medical regimen; "additional acts"
11. rules; regulations
12. American Nurses Association; National Council of State Boards of Nursing
13. rules; regulations
14. revocation of license; restrictions on license
15. endorsement
16. NCLEX-RN
17. computerized adaptive testing
18. prevent exploitation of foreign nurses; ensure the safety of the public
19. the American Nurses Association; AWHONN; AACCN (and many others, listed in the Table 4 of the textbook)
20. master's degree

True-False Questions

1. T
2. F
3. T
4. T
5. T
6. T
7. T
8. F
9. T
10. F
11. F
12. F
13. T
14. T
15. F
16. T
17. T
18. T
19. T
20. T
21. F
22. F
23. F
24. F
25. F

Matching Questions

A.
1. b
2. c
3. d
4. a
5. e

B.
1. e
2. b
3. a
4. c
5. d

Multiple-Choice Questions

1. a
2. d
3. c
4. a
5. c
6. a
7. b
8. a
9. a
10. c
11. c
12. c
13. c
14. c
15. b
16. d
17. a
18. a
19. b
20. b
21. c
22. d
23. b
24. b
25. d
26. d
27. a
28. b
29. c
30. d
31. b
32. d

Chapter 5 - Legal Responsibilities for Practice

Fill-In-The-Blank Questions

1. ethics
2. Law
3. common
4. statutory
5. statutory
6. common
7. criminal
8. civil
9. negligence
10. malpractice
11. defamation of character
12. Privileged communication
13. Liability insurance
14. claims occurred insurance coverage
15. respondent superior
16. charitable immunity
17. nonprofit health providers
18. (Any one) critical; fault-finding; demanding; angry

19. (Any one) give excellent care; communicate effectively; identify psychosocial needs and respond appropriately; demonstrate a caring attitude
20. deposition

True-False Questions

1. F
2. F
3. F
4. T
5. T
6. T
7. F
8. F
9. T
10. F
11. F
12. F
13. T

Matching Questions

1. f
2. c
3. e
4. d
5. a
6. b

Multiple-Choice Questions

1. b
2. c
3. d
4. a
5. b

6. d
7. c
8. c
9. a
10. c
11. b
12. d
13. b
14. b
15. b
16. d
17. a

Chapter 6 - Ethical Concerns in Nursing Practice

Fill-In-The-Blank Quesitons

1. Values clarification
2. rights
3. beneficence
4. autonomy
5. justice
6. Fidelity
7. ethical theory
8. utilitarianism
9. social justice
10. collegial
11. paternalism, authoritarianism
12. slander
13. pilfering
14. collect adequate information

True-False Questions

1. T
2. T
3. F

4. F
5. F
6. F
7. T
8. F
9. F
10. F
11. T
12. T
13. F
14. T
15. F
16. F
17. T
18. T
19. F
20. T

Matching Questions

A.
1. c
2. e
3. a
4. b
5. d

B.
1. d
2. a
3. c
4. b

Multiple-Choice Questions

1. c
2. d
3. d
4. c

5. b
6. d
7. b
8. c
9. b
10. a
11. a
12. c
13. a
14. a
15. d
16. c
17. d
18. a
19. d
20. a
21. c
22. b
23. b
24. a
25. b
26. d
27. a
28. d
29. c
30. b

Chapter 7 - Bioethical Issues in Health Care

Fill-In-The-Blank Questions

1. Bioethics
2. prevented conception
3. 1965
4. age of consent
5. mature minor

6. therapeutic abortion
7. *Roe v. Wade*
8. amniocentesis
9. eugenics
10. surrogate motherhood
11. homologous
12. *Black's Law Dictionary*
13. good death
14. positive
15. scarce medical resources

True-False Questions

1. T
2. F
3. T
4. F
5. F
6. T
7. T
8. F
9. T
10. F
11. F
12. T
13. T
14. T
15. F
16. F
17. F
18. T
19. F
20. T

Matching Questions

A.
1. c

2. d
3. e
4. a
5. b

B.
1. d
2. c
3. a
4. b

Multiple-Choice Questions

1. b
2. a
3. c
4. d
5. c
6. c
7. b
8. d
9. a
10. c
11. d
12. d
13. b
14. c
15. a
16. b
17. c
18. d
19. a
20. d
21. b
22. b
23. d
24. b

25. c
26. c
27. b
28. c
29. c
30. a

Chapter 8 - the Health Care Delivery System

Fill-In-The-Blank Questions

1. primary care provider
2. physician's assistants
3. therapist
4. health department
5. rural
6. caring
7. medicine
8. outside
9. diagnosis-related groups

True-False Questions

1. F
2. T
3. F
4. F
5. F
6. T
7. F
8. T

Multiple-Choice Questions

1. a
2. a
3. c
4. d
5. c
6. b
7. c
8. c
9. d
10. b
11. b
12. b
13. d
14. c
15. b
16. b
17. a
18. d
19. d
20. c
21. d
22. c
23. d

Chapter 9 - Collective Bargaining

Fill-In-The-Blank Questions

1. negotiating or bargaining
2. 1974
3. secret ballot
4. Horace Greeley
5. Wagner Act
6. Taft-Hartley Act; Labor Management Relations Act
7. collective bargaining
8. negotiating
9. collective action division
10. unfair labor practice

11. encourages membership in the union
12. binding arbitration
13. at an impasse; deadlocked
14. the cost involved or that it may result in a contract with which neither party is really pleased
15. financial remuneration; nonfinancial rewards; guidelines for grievances
16. writing; resolve
17. grievance
18. state nurses' associations
19. reinstatement privilege
20. strike
21. Concession bargaining
22. pay equity

True-False Questions

1. T
2. T
3. F
4. T
5. F
6. F
7. F
8. T
9. F
10. T
11. F
12. T
13. T
14. F
15. T
16. T
17. T
18. F
19. T
20. F
21. F
22. F
23. F
24. T

Matching Questions

A.
  1. c
  2. d
  3. b
  4. e
  5. a

B.
  1. d
  2. a
  3. e
  4. c
  5. b

C.
  1. d
  2. a
  3. c
  4. e
  5. b

Multiple-Choice Questions

1. a
2. c
3. b
4. c
5. a
6. b

7. c
8. d
9. a
10. a
11. a
12. b
13. c
14. b
15. d
16. d
17. c
18. b
19. b
20. a
21. a
22. a

Chapter 10 - the Political Process and Health Care

Fill-In-The-Blank Questions

1. (Any three) voting; keeping informed; supporting a candidate; telephone calls; telegrams; letters; working with an organization
2. construction; curriculum support
3. Medicare; Medicaid
4. maintain health and safety in the work place
5. promote health of pregnant women, mothers, infants, and children
6. authorization; appropriation
7. Appropriations
8. ANA-PAC

TRUE-FALSE QUESTIONS

1. T
2. F
3. F
4. F
5. T
6. F
7. F
8. F
9. F
10. F
11. T
12. T
13. T
14. T
15. F
16. F
17. T
18. T
19. T
20. T

Multiple-Choice Questions

1. b
2. a
3. d
4. a
5. c
6. c
7. d
8. a
9. a
10. a
11. a
12. d

13. b
14. a
15. a
16. a
17. d
18. b
19. d
20. c
21. d
22. d
23. b

Chapter 11 - Beginning Your Career as a Nurse

Fill-In-The-Blank Questions

1. greater
2. Council of Associate Degree Program (CADP) of the NLN
3. licensed practical nurses; associate degree nurses; baccalaureate nurses
4. (Any three) theoretical background; use of nursing process; recognition of own abilities and limitations; understanding of record-keeping; understanding of and commitment to a work ethic
5. chronic stress related to one's job, identified by feelings of hopelessness and powerlessness
6. references
7. Men
8. four

True-False Questions

1. F
2. T
3. T
4. T
5. F
6. T
7. T
8. F
9. T
10. F
11. T
12. F
13. T
14. T
15. F
16. T
17. T
18. F
19. F
20. T
21. F
22. T
23. F
24. F
25. T
26. T

Multiple-Choice Questions

1. a
2. b
3. b
4. a
5. c
6. d
7. c

8. a
9. b
10. c
11. a
12. a
13. a
14. d
15. c
16. b
17. b
18. d
19. b
20. a
21. b
22. c
23. b

Chapter 12 - Understanding Nursing Employment Settings

Fill-In-The-Blank Questions

1. days
2. Pennsylvania
3. mentally ill
4. 30
5. board
6. administrator
7. medical staff
8. director or assistant administrator for Nursing Services
9. mission statement
10. broad or wide
11. tall
12. team
13. primary
14. clinical ladder

True-False Questions

1. T
2. F
3. F
4. T
5. F
6. T
7. F
8. T
9. T
10. F
11. T
12. F
13. T
14. T
15. F
16. F
17. F
18. F
19. F
20. T

Multiple-Choice Questions

1. c
2. b
3. b
4. a
5. c
6. b
7. b
8. a
9. d
10. a
11. b

Chapter 13 - *Organizations for and about Nursing*

Fill-In-The-Blank Questions

1. economic
2. state associations
3. ANA
4. recruiting minorities into nursing and retaining them
5. promote quality nursing care
6. individuals and organizations interested in promoting quality nursing care
7. NLN
8. NLN
9. voluntary
10. American Academy of Nursing
11. Fellow of the American Academy of Nursing
12. ANA-PAC

True-False Questions

1. T
2. T
3. F
4. F
5. F
6. T
7. T
8. T
9. T
10. T
11. F
12. T
13. F
14. F
15. T
16. T
17. F
18. F

Multiple-Choice Questions

1. b
2. a
3. d
4. d
5. b
6. d
7. a
8. c
9. b
10. a
11. d
12. c
13. d
14. b